Felipe de Souza Cardoso

Sorbitol in Lactation

Felipe de Souza Cardoso

Sorbitol in Lactation

clinical, nutritional and toxicological effects

ScienciaScripts

Cover image: www.ingimage.com

This book is a translation from the original published under ISBN 978-613-9-61786-9.

Publisher:
Sciencia Scripts
is a trademark of
Dodo Books Indian Ocean Ltd. and OmniScriptum S.R.L publishing group

120 High Road, East Finchley, London, N2 9ED, United Kingdom
Str. Armeneasca 28/1, office 1, Chisinau MD-2012, Republic of Moldova, Europe
Printed at: see last page
ISBN: 978-620-7-70126-1

SUMMARY

ACKNOWLEDGMENTS

To my advisor, Professor Israel Felzenszwalb, for welcoming me to the Environmental Mutagenesis Laboratory (Labmut), believing in my project, guiding me over the last two years and contributing to my development as a researcher and teacher.

To my advisor, Professor Claudia Aiub, for all the dedication, seriousness, experience and competence applied to the development of this project.

To my friends and fellow professionals at Labmut, I would like to express my immense gratitude. Words cannot describe how important you have been in this phase of challenges, overcoming obstacles... You were my closest family.

Some people, in particular, Carlos, Andréia, Vanessa, Claudinha, Raphael, Elisa, Chico, Alessandras, Rafinha, Juliana, I would like to thank for all the hours and days dedicated to the animal surgeries and other important stages of my project.

To Professor Patricia Lisboa, for stimulating my methodological acuity, allowing me to evolve as a student, researcher, teacher and clinical professional. I am even more grateful for her contribution to the revision of this work.

To the Graduate Program in Clinical and Experimental Pathophysiology, for having believed in my project.

To the dear professors, members of the evaluation panel, thank you very much for accepting and dedicating your time to collaborating on my project.

To my friend Ellen Santos, for all the teachings, hours of venting, crying, strength and positive energy passed on during this journey.

To my dear colleagues in the Department of Biochemistry, who allowed me to use the microscope for many days and hours, essential for the completion of this work.

The Department of Pharmacology, which provided me with the space and conditions to carry out the liver perfusions and other stages of the surgeries.

The Experimental Surgery Laboratory (LCE), which allowed me to house the animals during the lactation period.

To the staff and biotherapists at LCE, thank you very much for all your concern and care for my animals.

To the central vivarium of the Federal University of Rio de Janeiro (UFRJ), which provided me with all the animals for the development of this project.

To the animals and bacteria for allowing me to carry out the project.

To Professor Clàudia Saunders and the Maternity School of UFRJ, for "introducing" me to sorbitol and helping to stimulate my research.

I would like to thank my family, both present and absent, for not letting me give up, for their strength and positive energy. I love you all!

In particular, I would like to thank my mother for having accompanied me from afar, for having been my father and mother, for giving me all the strength and conditions I needed to live and be here.

To Rodrigo, for his understanding during the long periods of absence dedicated to this work.

To the friends who, in some way, accompanied me and, therefore, are also part of this achievement.

To CNPq, FAPERJ and CAPES for all their support and investment.

"What a strange fate befalls us mortals! Each one of

we are here for a season, for what purpose we don't
know [...]. The ideals that have illuminated my path and

have repeatedly renewed my courage to face
life with courage: Goodness, Beauty and Truth."

Albert Einstein

SUMMARY

CARDOSO, Felipe de Souza. Effects of maternal sorbitol intake during lactation on the nutritional, biochemical and toxicological profile of breastfed offspring, 2013. 77f - Faculty of Medical Sciences, Rio de Janeiro State University, Rio de Janeiro, 2013.

Sorbitol is a polyol found in special-purpose products, such as *diet* and *light,* consumed by people who want to achieve a slim aesthetic standard. Within this context, Iactating women are major consumers, aiming to return to their pre-gestational weight as quickly as possible. Due to the lack of data on the metabolic consequences of excessive consumption of these types of products, especially during this critical period of development (pregnancy and lactation), the aim of this study was to evaluate the possible effects of maternal intake of sorbitol during lactation on the nutritional, biochemical and toxicological profiles of breastfed offspring. The Salmonella/microsome test was initially used for mutagenic and cytotoxic evaluation with strains of *S. enterica* serovar Typhimurium (TA97, TA98, TA100, TA102, TA104 and TA1535). We checked the mutation reversal capacity (I.M.) and survival (%) when in contact with sorbitol at different concentrations (0.4; 4; 40; 400; 4000 and 5000 µg/plate). The results were considered positive for M.I. values ≥ 2.0. Lactating *wistar* rats (6 per experimental group), each with 6 pups, were given sorbitol (0.00015 mg/g/day; 0.0015 mg/g/day and 0.15 mg/g/day) for the first 14 days of lactation. During this period, we evaluated the biometrics of the mothers and offspring, feed consumption and the mothers' water intake. After lactation, the mother rats were milked and, together with the offspring, sacrificed by cardiac puncture for whole blood collection. The offspring's livers were perfused to obtain hepatocytes in primary culture at the end of 14 days of lactation. The femurs of the offspring were removed to obtain bone marrow. The blood biochemistry of the offspring (glucose, triglycerides, total cholesterol, LDL, total protein, albumin, ALT, AST, total and ionized calcium) was analyzed, as well as the biochemistry of the milked milk (triglycerides). The micronucleus tests on bone marrow and hepatocytes, as well as the Comet test on whole blood, were used for genotoxic and cytotoxic evaluation, in accordance with OECD guidelines. The results showed that, at lower concentrations (0.00015 and 0.0015 mg/g), sorbitol induced weight gain, especially at the lowest concentration (0.00015 mg/g), and alterations in the blood lipid profile at all concentrations. The amounts of triglyceride in the milk varied depending on the dose ingested, reduced at the highest concentration (0.15 mg/g) and increased at the lowest (0.00015 mg/g). The highest concentration (0.15 mg/g) resulted in weight loss in mothers and offspring, a decrease in total visceral proteins, albumin and an increase in liver enzymes (ALT and AST) in the offspring. The results of the *Salmonella/microsome* test did not indicate mutagenicity; however, there was a dose-dependent relationship between dose and Mutagenicity Index (M.I.). Both tests, bone marrow micronuclei and hepatocytes, showed statistically significant dose-dependent cytotoxicity compared to the control group, corroborating the genotoxicity of the Comet test and the dose dependence found in the *Salmonella/microsome test.* At lower concentrations, there seems to be modulation of lipogenic pathways, while at higher concentrations, toxicity seems to hinder these changes, inducing the opposite effect. We conclude that excessive consumption of sorbitol could result in metabolic and toxicological alterations in breastfeeding women and infants, even though it is considered safe by the FDA and ANVISA.

Keywords: sorbitol, lactation, obesity, dyslipidemia, hepatotoxicity,

Salmonella/microsome, micronucleus, comet test.

1. INTRODUCTION

1.1 Chemical and physico-chemical characteristics of sorbitol

Sorbitol, 1,2,3,4,5,6-hexanehexol ($C_6H_{14}O_6$), molecular weight 182.17 g/mol, is a polyol widely found in nature (Figure 1), mainly in some foods (Table 1), such as apples, pears, peaches, plums, cherries, seaweed and fermented beverages in quantities not sufficient for commercial extraction, and its industrial production is therefore made from sucrose and starch, by hydrolysis followed by catalytic hydrogenation (Figure 2), the method with the highest yield (LEE *et al.*, 1994; CÂNDIDO and CAMPOS, 1996; ADA, 2004; TORLONI *et al.*, 2007; MUIR *et al.*, 2009; FDA, 2012).

Table 1 - Amount (g) of sorbitol per 100 g of food.

Food	Sorbitol (g/100g)
Apple	0,2-1,0
Apple juice	0,3-1,0
Cherry	1,4-2,1
Grapes	0,2
Pear	1,2-3,5
Pear juice	1,1-2,6
Plum	0,3-2,8
Strawberry	< 0,1
Melao	1,0-5,0
Tomato	< 0,1

Source: adapted from HALLFRISCH *et al.* (1990)

It is a stereoisomer of mannitol (Figure 2), which is also widely used in the food industry, differing in the hydroxyl of carbon two, thus presenting alterations in solubility, hygroscopicity, laxative potential and calorie content (2.4Kcal/g).

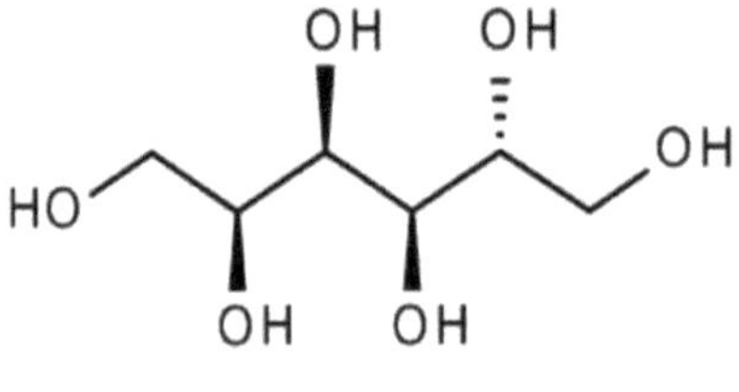

Figura 1: sorbitol structural formula. Source: MERCK.

Its physico-chemical characteristics allow it to be highly refreshing (heat of dissolution 26.6Kcal/kg), chemically, bacteriologically and thermally stable (melting point between 96 and

97°C), non-volatile, with intramolecular water elimination only when exposed to a minimum temperature of 160°C for long periods.

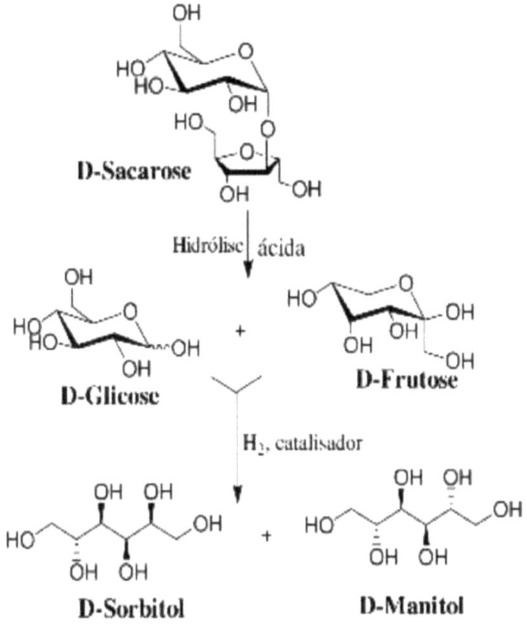

D-Sacarose
Hidrólise ácida
D-Glicose + D-Frutose
H_2, catalisador
D-Sorbitol + D-Manitol

Figura 2: Chemical structure and industrial synthesis of D-Sorbitol and D-Manitol.

Source: OLIVEIRA *et al.*, 2009.

2.2 Marketing of sorbitol and products containing it

Sorbitol is marketed as syrup (70%) or powder (sorbitans and sorbates). It is water-soluble, thermostable, widely found in industrialized products for dietary purposes (sweeteners, cereal bars, honey buns, jams, chewing gums, cookies, chocolates, soft drinks, etc.) and endogenously synthesized from the hydrogenation of glucose, a reaction catalyzed by the enzyme aldose reductase, an NADPH-dependent oxidoreductase. When used by the food industry, it acts as a body agent, carrier, thickener, antifreeze, chelating agent, stabilizer, humectant, plasticizer, sweetener, improving the aftertaste of other sweeteners such as saccharin, fixing aromas and flavours and having a sweetness of between 0.5 and 0.7% compared to sucrose. (LEE *et al.*, 1994; CÂNDIDO & CAMPOS, 1996; ADA, 2004; TORLONI *et al.*, 2007; MUIR *et al.,* 2009).

2.3 Legislation for the use of sorbitol in Brazil and worldwide

In 1959, the USA already included sorbitol as a *GRAS* substance, with a maximum of 7% being used in foods for dietary purposes. In 1961 it became a nutrient and/or dietary supplement and was regulated as an additive (15g/portion and maximum intake of 40g/day). This was reflected in Decree 55.871/65 and Resolution 9/79 of the Food Technical Chamber, which authorized the use of sorbitol without limits in soft drinks, other beverages and foods for dietary purposes, as a sweetener, with the requirement to respect Good Manufacturing Practices (GMP). As these documents are revised periodically, in 1974 the FDA maintained the *GRAS status* for sorbitol, within Good Manufacturing Practice, but set some maximum limits, as in some European countries (Portugal and Spain). The World Health Organization (WHO), since 1982, has also not established an adequate intake, as it considers it chemically, biochemically and toxicologically safe for human consumption, even in the face of the maximum quantities declared in some European countries (25 - 40g/day).

In Brazil, the National Health Surveillance Agency (ANVISA) was created by Law 9.782/99, which defined its organizational structure, management model, positions, functions, assets and revenues with the institutional purpose of promoting the protection of the health of the population, through the sanitary control of the production and marketing of products and services subject to sanitary surveillance. By regulating sorbitol as a food additive and technology adjuvant in the food industry, the latter subjected products containing it to supervision, given the need for use and safety against potential toxicological risks. According to ANVISA (1997), additives, any ingredient intentionally added to food, without the purpose of nourishing it and with the aim of modifying its physical, chemical, biological or sensory characteristics, during the manufacture, processing, treatment, packaging, storage, transportation or handling of the food, were permitted and divided according to maximum limits and functions for technological purposes. Interested parties had to submit a proposal with proof of safety, technological need, proposed limit, estimated intake and internationally recognized references, which was evaluated by committees of experts from the World Health Organization (WHO) and the Food and Agriculture Organization (FAO), known as the Joint FAO/WHO Expert Committee on Food Additives (JECFA, 2012), updated by ANVISA itself and agreements within MERCOSUR. Approval of a food additive in Brazil would require international positions from the European Union (*Codex Alimentarius*, 2012) and the United States of America (FDA - *Food and Drug Administration,* 2012), criteria established by current Brazilian legislation, ANVISA ordinance 540 (1997), MERCOSUR/GMC/RES 52/98.

Their use in foods and drinks for weight control, controlled sugar intake, sugar restriction and others with complementary nutritional information was considered safe for human consumption, according to ANVISA in 2008, and the industry was therefore allowed to use the quantity required for the ideal product, This resulted in the publication of Collegiate Board Resolution 27 (ANVISA,

2010a), in which additives and adjuvants are exempt from mandatory registration, with manufacturers being responsible for communicating the initial procedures required.

However, we know that there is still a lack of specific studies involving the use of this polyol, especially during critical periods of development, such as pregnancy and lactation, which has led the Ministry of Health (MS) to establish its careful use among lactating women (ANVISA, 2010b).

In April 2012, the code of federal regulations on sorbitol was revised by the FDA, which waived some previous sanctions, but kept it as *GRAS* and some maximum limits for food products (FDA, 2012).

2.4 Toxicological evaluation of food additives in Brazil and the world

In Brazil, ANVISA is the regulatory body responsible for protecting the health of the population through the sanitary control of the production and marketing of products, using international references such as the OECD guidelines. The OECD is a global reference organization that promotes the gathering of guidelines for the evaluation of chemical substances, using standardized scientific methods, which characterize possible risks to the health of the population.

The OECD presents proposals for genotoxic tests, both *in vitro* and *in vivo,* which are important for evaluating mutagenic, cytotoxic and genotoxic properties, especially when it comes to human consumption. The bacterial reverse mutation test is part of the first line of tests, as it has been shown that many compounds that are positive in these protocols also behave as such in eukaryotes. In addition, they are quick and inexpensive (MOHN, 1981; PURCHASE, 1982; MARON & AMES, 1983; MORTHELMANS & ZEIGER, 2000).

After this first protocol, two more tests are required: an *in vitro* cytogenetic test to assess chromosomal damage, such as the micronucleus test, and another *in vivo* test to assess chromosomal damage in rodent hematopoietic cells. As an alternative option, the OECD indicates the bacterial reverse mutation test and an *in vivo* test with rodent hematopoietic cells and hepatocytes (OECD 471, 474, 1997; OECD 487, 2010). The micronucleus test, both *in vitro* and *in vivo, is* used for genotoxic evaluation with the formation of small pieces of membrane-bound DNA, mainly in micronucleated polychromatic erythrocytes from bone marrow (OECD 474, 1997).

The results are interpreted and analyzed to determine possible risks in human consumption. Generally, when no genotoxic effects have been demonstrated in two *in vivo* tests, the risk to human health is considered to be exempt (OECD 471, 474, 1997; OECD 487, 2010).

2.5 Epidemiological indicators and dietary profile of the population

Epidemiological, pre-clinical, clinical and experimental studies indicate a correlation between exposure to nutritional, hormonal and environmental factors during critical periods of development, such as pregnancy and lactation, and the onset of morbidities in adult life, such as obesity, insulin resistance, diabetes, dyslipidemia, cancer, etc. This phenomenon is known as metabolic programming or ontogenetic plasticity (MOURA *et al.*, 2008; CEDERROTH & NEF, 2009).

Currently, with changes in morbidity and mortality patterns, obesity is gaining prominence, along with other chronic diseases, resulting in an increase in the consumption of sweeteners and special-purpose products that claim to provide a sweet taste without increasing calorie intake (CARMO *et al.*, 2003; LEVY-COSTA *et al.,* 2005; CASTRO & FRANCO, 2002). Polyols, which are sugar substitutes, have gained prominence for having slower passive absorption when compared to fructose and glucose, a fact which justifies their lower calorie intake and increased demand for *diet* and *light* products (DRUZIAN *et al.*, 2005). According to the Family Budget Survey (IBGE, 2009), the consumption of fruit, vegetables and legumes by more than 90% of the Brazilian population is still below the levels recommended by the Ministry of Health (400g), reflecting an increase in the consumption of industrialized products containing large quantities of additives such as sorbitol (SOUZA *et al.*, 2011).

Within this context, we have seen an increase in the prevalence of obesity in pregnant women, as shown by data from NHANES (2004) in which 28.9% of women (2039 years) had a Body Mass Index (BMI) above 30 kg/m^2 , corroborating Brazilian data from the Surveillance of Risk and Protective Factors for Chronic Diseases by Telephone Survey (VIGITEL), provided by the Brazilian Institute of Geography and Statistics (IBGE) on the growth of overweight, dependent age group. According to the Institute of Medicine (IOM, 2009), the recommended weight gain during pregnancy is based on the pre-pregnancy Body Mass Index (BMI) and most pregnant women gain excessive weight during this period, either because they already have a high pre-pregnancy BMI or because of uncontrolled weight gain during this period, and it is not uncommon to find breastfeeding women with the consequences of acquired excess weight, seeking solutions to return to their ideal weight (ROCHA *et al.*, 2005; STULBACH *et al.*, 2007; DEIERLEIN *et al.*, 2010; RONNBERG & NILSON, 2010). At the same time, there has been a growth in the beauty and value of models proposed by fashion segments, around the perfect (slim) body and motivated by the desire to achieve the aesthetic standards demanded by the current culture, without considering aspects related to health, women submit to successive restrictive diets and excessive use of sweeteners (TORLONI *et al.*, 2007; RENWICK & MOLINARY, 2010). An explosion of scientific publications between the end of the 20th century and the beginning of the 21st century highlighted the singularity of the construction of beauty in our culture as an obsession and, today, the indiscriminate consumption of weight control products and the possible repercussions of these compounds at various stages of life, including critical periods of development (WITT & SCHNEIDER, 2011; BRUGNERA *et al.,* 2012).

2.6 Absorption, bioavailability, pathways, possible metabolic and toxicological consequences

It is known that there is no described active transport mechanism for sorbitol across the enterocyte membrane in the small intestine, but it is carried out by passive diffusion, according to the concentration gradient, using the same transporter as fructose, GLUT 5, located in the apical membrane. The absorption limit of this polyol can reach 79%, at which point its excretion is considered negligible, going to the liver and being efficiently metabolized by dehydrogenation, through the enzymatic action of sorbitol dehydrogenase, an enzyme dependent on zinc and NAD (Nicotinamide Adenine Dinucleotide), which catalyzes the reaction synthesizing fructose and its subsequent metabolic pathways (BARREIROS *et al.*, 2005). Blood and cellular levels of sorbitol can also increase independently of direct intake, through increased sugar consumption or in special situations, such as insulin resistance and diabetes mellitus, all of which result in an increase in blood glucose, with D-Glucose being converted to D-Sorbitol by the action of aldose reductase (BARRETOS *et al.*, 2005), a natural occurrence in diabetics, in whom glucose, independent of insulin, enters the liver, easily following the polyol pathway. In the nervous system, also independent of insulin, it can result in cataracts, diabetic polyneuropathy, retinal and renal microangiopathy (BOSCO *et al.*, 2005). Fructose can be phosphorylated by fructokinase, generating dihydroxyketone phosphate, glyceraldehyde and glycerol, which favor lipogenic pathways and metabolic consequences contrary to those mentioned above (Figure 3), such as hypertriglyceridemia, hypercholesterolemia, adipogenesis, with the possibility of NASH (BANTLE, 1991; SHAFRIR, 1991; CHAVES *et al.,* 2012). It is not considered toxic, mutagenic, teratogenic or carcinogenic in previous studies, however, in excessive doses (5-70g/day) it could cause abdominal discomfort, increased diuresis, laxative effect and cellular events such as apoptotic and changes in intracellular redox potential (WILLIAM,1989; ASNAGHI *et al.*, 2003; JAUNIAUX et al., 2005; SAUNDERS *et al.,* 2010).

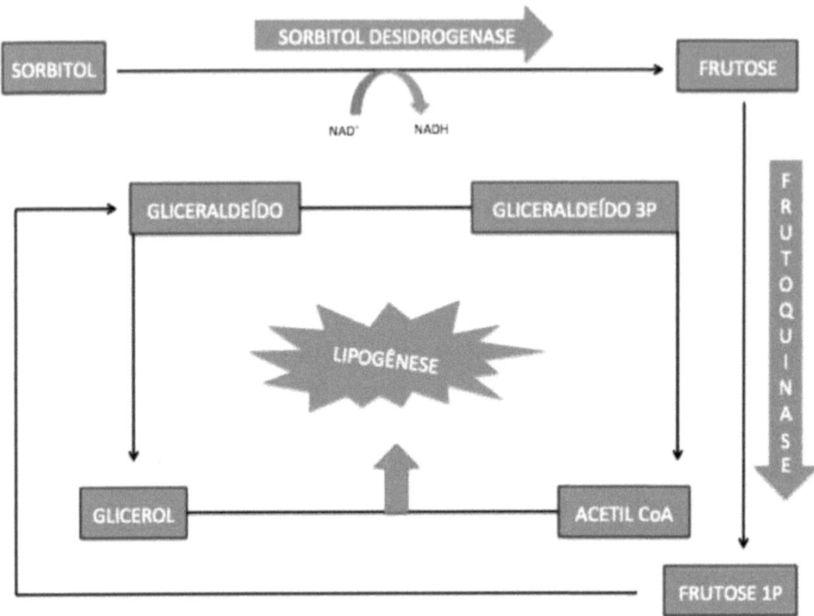

Figura 3: possible metabolic pathways between sorbitol and lipogenesis. Source: adapted from BARREIROS *et al*. (2005).

2. OBJECTIVES

2.1 General objective

To evaluate the effects of maternal intake of different doses of sorbitol in the first 14 days of lactation on nutritional, biochemical and toxicological parameters in lactating *wistar* rats and their offspring.

2.2 Specific objectives

- To evaluate the mutagenic and cytotoxic capacity of sorbitol, at different concentrations, through the bacterial reverse mutation test (*Salmonella/microsome*) in strains (TA97, TA98, TA100, TA102, TA104 and TA1535) of *Salmonella enterica* serovar Typhimurium, in the presence and absence of metabolic activation.
- To evaluate the effects of maternal intake of different doses of sorbitol during lactation in relation to the weight, feed consumption and water intake of the mothers.
- To evaluate the effects of maternal consumption of different doses of sorbitol during lactation on the amount of triglycerides present in the breast milk of lactating *wistar* rats.
- To evaluate the effects of maternal sorbitol intake during lactation in relation to the weight and length of lactating offspring.
- To evaluate the effects of maternal consumption of sorbitol during lactation on the biochemical profile of infant offspring.
- To evaluate whether there are possible cytotoxic and genotoxic effects in the offspring of lactating *wistar* rats that ingest sorbitol in different concentrations.

3. MATERIAL AND METHODS

3.1 Ethics committee

The project was submitted to the Ethics Committee for the Care and Use of Experimental Animals and certified under protocol number CEUA/064/2012 (appendix 1).

3.2 Toxicological evaluation in prokaryotes

3.2.1 Induction of bacterial reverse mutation (Salmonella/microsome/Ames test)

The Ames test in prokaryotes, as well as the micronucleus and comet assays in eukaryotes, are recognized by international regulatory bodies and are therefore used to assess mutagenicity, cytotoxicity and genotoxicity, respectively, for various chemical agents (MORTELMANS & ZEIGER, 2000).

The bacterial reverse mutation assay is able to detect the mutagenicity of substances in prokaryotes. The assay often uses exogenous metabolization, through a microsomal fraction known as S9 mix (Molecular Toxicology Inc. USA), which mimics the eukaryotic system. This is presented as a homogenate of the liver of male *Sprague-Dawley* rats, which are treated with biphenyl-polychlorinate, a stimulant of the metabolizing enzyme system. To prepare 50 mL of the S9 mix (4% v/v), 19.75 mL of distilled water was used; 25.0 mL of sodium phosphate buffer (0.2 M; pH 7.4); 2.0 mL of NADP solution (0.1M); 0.25 mL of glucose-6-phosphate (1M); 1 mL of $MgCl_2$-KCl salts (0.15 M) and 2.0 mL of lyophilized S9, which was reconstituted in distilled water (MARON & AMES, 1983; OECD 471, 1997; MORTELMANS & ZEIGER, 2000).

The strains of the bacterium *S. enterica* serovar Typhimurium used had substitutions, additions or deletions of base pairs in various *loci of* their genes, resulting in a deficiency in the synthesis of the amino acid histidine. The test verified the ability of the mutations to be reversed when in contact with sorbitol at different concentrations (0.4; 4; 40; 400; 4000; 5000 µg/plate). Four strains of *Salmonella enterica* serovar Typhimurium were used (TA97, TA98, TA100, TA102, TA104 and TA1535), as shown in Table 4 (MARON & AMES, 1983; MORTELMANS & ZEIGER, 2000).

Salmonella enterica serovar Typhimurium strain TA97 has a mutation (addition of a GC base pair) at the *hisD6610 locus*, and we have identified substances capable of deleting this addition and restoring the reading frame. The mutation (addition or deletion of the GC pair) in strain TA98 is located at the *hisD3052 locus*, which is important for the synthesis of the histidinol dehydrogenase enzyme. The mutation (substitution of the AT base pair for GC) in the *his* G46 *locus of* strain TA100 replaces the amino acid leucine with proline, leading to a deficiency in the synthesis of an important enzyme in the histidine pathway. The TA102 strain has an extra base pair in the *hisG428 locus*, which was inserted with the pAQ1 plasmid, conferring resistance to tetracycline. Strain TA104 has a mutation in the *hisG46 locus* and can reverse all six base pair combinations by transitions/transversions. Strain TA1535, like strain TA100, has the amino acid leucine replaced by proline.

Insertion of a base pair by plasmid is another mechanism for additional mutations, which may account for the bacteria's ability to respond to sorbitol exposure. The *uvrB* gene is deleted in strains TA97, TA98, TA100, TA104 and TA1535 leading to a deficiency in the nucleotide excision repair system, resulting in increased sensitivity in the detection of mutagens, as well as deletion of the system responsible for biotin synthesis. All the strains used (TA97, TA98, TA100, TA102, TA104 and TA1535) have a mutation in the *rfa* gene, which is important in the synthesis of Hpopolysaccharides (LPS), which behave as constituents of the cell wall of gram-negative bacteria, increasing their permeability to large molecules. Plasmids (pKM101 and pAQ1) are also used to increase bacterial sensitivity to possible test substances. The former increases the sensitivity of the system in detecting mutagenic substances by increasing the *error-prone* DNA repair pathway and selects ampicillin-resistant bacteria. The second increases the sites targeted by the test substances and provides resistance to the antibiotic tetracycline.

The positive controls, both in the presence and absence of metabolization, were used according to MARON & AMES (1983) and MORTELMANS & ZEIGER (2000), all shown in Table 2. As water diluted all the samples, we considered it as a negative control.

Table 2: positive controls in the presence and absence of metabolization.

	S9 +	S9 -
TA97	Amino Anthracene (1.0 μg/plate)	4 COD * (1.0 μg/plate)
TA98	Amino Anthracene (1.0 μg/plate)	4 COD * (1.0 μg/plate)
TA100	Amino Anthracene (1.0 μg/plate)	Sodium azide (1.0 μg/plate)
TA102	Benzopyrene (50 μg/plate)	Mitomycin C (0.5 μg/plate)
TA104	Amino Anthracene (1.0 μg/plate)	Mitomycin C (0.5 μg/plate)
TA1535	Amino Anthracene (1.0 μg/plate)	4 COD * (1.0 μg/plate)

* 4 NQO (4-Nitroquinoline 1- oxide)

Source: MARON & AMES (1983); MORTELMANS & ZEIGER (2000).

Aliquots (100 μL) of bacterial cultures in stationary phase (2.0 x 109 cells/mL) were obtained from *S. enterica* serovar Typhimurium strains (TA97, TA98, TA100, TA102, TA104 and TA1535). These were pre-incubated (20 min., 37°C, 120 rpm) in test tubes with 100 μL of sorbitol samples at various concentrations (0.4; 4; 40; 400; 4000; 5000μg/plate). Subsequently, 500 μL of sodium phosphate buffer (0.2 mM pH 7.4) was added, for the absence of metabolization, or 500 μL of S9 mix, for the presence of metabolization. We removed 10 µL of the suspension for a survival test, carried out in parallel with the mutagenicity test, and added 2.0 mL of topagar (0.7% agar; 0.6% NaCl; 50 µM L-histidine; 50 µM biotin; pH 7.4; 45°C). This mixture was plated on minimal agar medium [1.5% agar; 10x Vogel-Bonner medium (10 g/L $MgSO_4.7H_2O$; 100 g/L $C_6H_8O_7.H_2O$; 500 g/L K_2HPO_4; 175 g/L $Na(NH_4)HPO_4.4H_2O$)], containing 2% glucose). The plates were incubated for 72 hours at 37°C and, after this period, the colonies (number of revertants - CR) were counted. After counting, the CR of the samples was divided by the CR of the negative control and the result of this ratio was considered to be the mutagenicity index (M.I.). We consider M.I. results equal to or greater than 2.0 to be mutagenic (AIUB *et al.*, 2004).

The survival test was carried out in parallel with the mutagenicity test to avoid possible interpretation problems. Therefore, from 10 µL of the pre-incubated mixture, a serial dilution (10^{-7}) was carried out in 0.9% NaCl, ensuring a good count. A final aliquot (100 µL), after the dilutions, was added to a petri dish prepared with Louria-Bertani medium (0.8% nutrients; 0.5% NaCl and 1.5% Agar), incubated (37°C / 24 h.) and counted immediately afterwards. The result is considered cytotoxic when the "survival rate" is below 70% compared to the negative control (AIUB *et al.*, 2004).

Table 3: Mutation sites and genotype of *Salmonella enterica* serovar Typhimurium strains.

LINEAGE	REVERSE	(*uvrB/Bio*)	(LPS)	PLASMiDEOS	Mutated *loci*
TA97	Deletion (G-C)	Deletion	*rfa*	pKM101	hisD6610
TA98	Addition or deletion (G-C)	Deletion	*rfa*	pKM101	hisD3052
TA100	Substitutions (G-C for T-A)	Deletion	*rfa*	pKM101	hisG46
TA102	Substitutions (T-A for G-C)	-	*rfa*	pKM101 / pAQ1	hisG428
TA104	Transition/Transversion (TAA)	Deletion	*rfa*	-	hisG428
TA1535	Substitutions (GAG/CTC for GGG/CCC)	Deletion	*rfa*	-	hisG46

Source: MORTELMANS & ZEIGER (2000).

3.3 Maternal sorbitol intake during lactation

3.3.1 Treatment and monitoring of animals in vivaria

Wistar rats were obtained in late pregnancy from the vivarium of the Federal University of Rio de Janeiro (UFRJ). We received them with information about their pre-gestational and current weights, at the time they were handed over. They were transported to the vivarium of the Experimental Surgery Laboratory (LCE) of the State University of Rio de Janeiro (UERJ), housed in individual cages and given water and feed *ad libitum*. On the day of birth, the number of pups and their sex were recorded for control and standardization, totaling six final pups for each mother, most of them males. They were all housed in separate boxes, resulting in four groups, each with six mothers and each mother with six chicks. The lactating rats were kept for 14 days in a controlled animal house (temperature and light/dark cycles), receiving commercial feed (17.35% protein; 52.12% carbohydrate; 7.64% lipid), water *ad libitum* during the day and sorbitol (0.00015 mg/g; 0.0015 mg/g and 0.15 mg/g) at night, from the first day of lactation. During the day, the rats received water *ad libitum and its* volume was identified in the late afternoon, between 5 and 6 p.m., before treatment (FIGUEIREDO *et al., 2009).* The experimental groups are: control (water); Sorbitol 1 (0.00015 mg/g); Sorbitol 2 (0.0015 mg/g) and Sorbitol 3 (0.15 mg/g).

3.3.2 Evaluation of weight, length, feed intake and water intake

During the follow-up period in the vivarium, mothers and offspring were weighed daily on an electronic scale. The length of the mothers, in centimeters, was checked on the first day of monitoring and the length of the offspring was checked daily, both using a standard tape measure. The feed intake of the mothers was checked daily by weighing the remainder obtained from the amount fed the previous day. Water intake was checked daily, using the remainder obtained from a 50 mL supply, using a small beaker, always in the late afternoon, between 5 and 6 p.m., before treatment.

3.3.3 Cardiac puncture, liver perfusion, sacrifice and primary hepatocyte culture

After 14 days of lactation under treatment, the mothers and pups, fasting overnight, were anaesthetized with pentobarbital 160 mg/Kg and underwent cardiac puncture, which was done at the same time as the liver perfusion procedure, so that the haemodynamics would not alter the procedure. The puncture was performed on the mothers and pups and the perfusion was performed on the pups only to obtain the *pool*. Each *pool* represented a mother from a given group. Whole blood was then obtained for subsequent biochemical analysis and toxicological evaluation using the comet test. Hepatocytes were obtained using the perfusion method proposed by KHADER *et al.* (2007) and AIUB *et al.* (2011) adapted in two stages. The animals were anaesthetized with pentobarbital (160 mg/kg) with posterior cannulation of the hepatic portal vein and perfusion with 75 mL of solution A (142 mM NaCl; 6.7 mM KCl; 10 mM HEPES, pH 7.4) for 5 min (15 mL/min). The liver was subsequently perfused with approximately 80 mL of solution C (9:1 of solution A and 5.7 mM $CaCl_2$, pH 7.4), containing 0.5 mg of collagenase/mL (40 mg of type I collagenase/fig from 14-day-old rats) for 8 min (10 mL/min). The perfused livers were carefully cut and placed in a closed, sterile flask containing 50 mL of solution A at 37°C for 10 min. The suspension was filtered through sterile gauze and the filtrate obtained was centrifuged at 500 rpm for 10 min. The supernatant was removed by inversion and the cells resuspended in Eagle's Minimal Essential Medium (MEM) 1.8 mM Ca^2 +, supplemented with 26.2 mM $NaHCO_3$; 1.2 mM pyruvate; 0.2 mM aspartic acid and 0.2 mM L- serine. The concentration of the stock suspension was obtained by counting in a Neubauer chamber using trypan blue (1:1). Viability was between 80 and 95% and 2.0 x 10^5 cells/mL were added to 60 mm plates and conditioned in a CO_2 oven (37°C; 5.0%) for 24 h (PERES, 2005; adapted from AIUB *et al.*, 2011; adapted from TURKETZ *et al.,* 2012).

3.4 Toxicological evaluation in eukaryotes

3.4.1 *In vivo* micronucleus and comet tests on mammalian cells

3.4.1.1 Micronucleus in hepatocytes

After 24 hours in the oven, the culture medium was removed from the plates and 5 mL of fresh, ice-cold fixative solution (3:1, Methanol: Acetic Acid) was added to each one, keeping it there for 5 min. Afterwards, the fixative was removed and 5 mL of Mc Ilvaine buffer was added [Solution A: Na_2 HPO_4 (0.2 M) in 1 L, Solution B: citric acid (0.1 M) in 300 mL of distilled water, mix solution B with solution A until pH 7.0, autoclave 121°C / 20 min), then remove and keep the plates open to dry. 2.5 mL of 4'6'- diamidino-2-phenylindol (DAPI) solution, diluted in Mc Ilvaine to a concentration of 300 mM, was added and kept in contact with the cells for 40 min. in a dark place. The DAPI was discarded in special waste and washed twice with Mc Ilvaine, the last wash being maintained for 3 min. The plates were dried in the dark and analyzed using fluorescence at 430 nm (OECD 487, 2010).

3.4.1.2 Micronucleus in bone marrow hematopoietic cells

Both femurs of the pups from each mother were removed, along with the excess tissue, with tweezers and scissors, and kept in RPMI medium (developed by the Roswell Park Memorial Institute), as a *pool,* until the time of the test. The ends of the bones were cut off, a 1 mL needle was inserted into the opening of one of the bone ends and the marrow was pushed into a centrifuge tube using Fetal Bovine Serum (FBS). The suspension obtained in FBS was centrifuged (1000 rpm/5 min) and the supernatant discarded by inversion. The sediment was resuspended in 0.5 mL of FBS again and two drops were dripped onto the edges of the slides used for reading. With the help of another slide, the smear was made and the slides were left to dry in the open air for 1 hour. After this period, the slides were placed in a staining vat with pure Giemsa for 3 minutes. They were then transferred to another vat with the dye diluted 1:6 in water. After these steps, the slides were rinsed in a vat of distilled water to remove excess dye. The support surfaces were wiped clean with paper towels and the slides were left in the open air for 24 hours to dry. The optical microscope was used for analysis, using 200 to 400 x magnification until a quality field was found to identify the cells and then the 1000 x objective (OECD 474, 1997).

3.4.1.3 Whole blood comet

The puppies' whole blood, approximately 1.0 mL, was obtained by cardiac puncture in a 1 mL syringe, separated by *pool for* each mother, at the same time as the liver perfusion. We worked with 5 slides for each *pool of* whole blood, referring to the 6 pups standardized for each mother, a representative component of an experimental group, made up of 5 mothers each. In total, we worked with three treated groups and one control group. The material was placed in microtubes containing 80 μL of heparin (5,000 IU/mL). In microcentrifuge tubes, 10 μL of whole blood was mixed with 120 μL of low melting point agarose (BPF 0.5% w/v), matured at 37±1°C, homogenized once and 120 μL was added to each slide (quintuplicate), previously prepared with normal melting point agarose (1.5% w/v). Immediately, the coverslip was placed on the slide, avoiding the formation of air bubbles. The slides were left in the refrigerator (4°C - 10°C) on racks for approximately 3 to 5 minutes to allow the agarose to polymerize. After this period, the coverslips were removed by gently sliding them over the agarose layer and immersing them in a container containing cell lysis solution [Solution 1: sodium chloride (2.5 M), disodium EDTA (100 mM), Tris (10 mM), sodium lauroyl sarcosinate (10 g), deionized water; Solution 2: triton X - 100 (1 mL),

dimethyl sulfoxide (DMSO) (10 mL) and lysis solution 1 to complete a final volume of 100 mL. The solution was prepared on the day of the test and kept cold (4°C to 10°C), protected from light. The slides were kept in the refrigerator for 1 week until the test was carried out. The steps were carried out in the absence of light to avoid further damage to the DNA. After this period, the slides were carefully removed from the lysis solution, removing excess solution from the edges and other parts. The slides were placed in the support of the horizontal electrophoresis vat, next to the positive pole (anode), as close as possible to each other, filling in the gaps with agarose-free slides. The vat (15 cm x 15 cm) was filled with 1,320 mL of fresh electrophoresis buffer [sodium hydroxide (10N); disodium EDTA (200 mM); deionized water], previously chilled in the fridge for at least 2 hours, until the liquid level completely covered the slides, avoiding bubbles on the agarose. The slides were kept in an alkaline lid for 40 min to allow the DNA to unwind and the different classes of DNA damage to be expressed. The power supply was switched on at 25 volts and the current set at 300 mA, slowly increasing and decreasing the level of the lid until the final setting was reached. The run lasted 25 min. Light was kept off during all stages. At the end of the electrophoretic run, the slides were carefully removed from the vat and placed in a support for neutralization, done by carefully covering all the slides with the neutralization cap [Tris X-100 (1mL); DMSO (10mL); NaCl (2.5M; 146.1g); disodium EDTA (100 mM; 37.2g); Tris (10 mM; 1.2g) and deionized water (qsp 1000 mL)], leaving for 5 min., repeating the neutralization process twice more. The slides were placed in a vat of absolute ethanol (99.2% to 99.5%) for 10 min. and dried at room temperature in a horizontal position for 24 hours. They were then kept in closed boxes for 1 week in a refrigerator (4°C to 10°C) and stained with DAPI immediately at the time of reading under the fluorescence microscope. The slides were analyzed at 400 x magnification, randomly selecting 50 cells per slide to assess the extent of DNA migration. The intensity of the comet tail was considered in four different classes (COLLINS, 2004): class 0 (no tail), class 1 (small tail), class 2 (large tail), class 3 (totally damaged, no defined comet head). The results were expressed as percentages and Arbitrary Units (AU), calculated according to the formula: UA=[(Mo x 0)+(M1 x 1)+(M2 x 2) + (M3 x 3)], where UA (number of arbitrary units), Mo (number of cells with damage class 0), M1 (number of cells with damage class 1), M2 (number of cells with damage class 2), M3 (number of cells with damage class 3). The assay is summarized in figure 4 (WASSON *et al.,* 2008; INCQS, 2009).

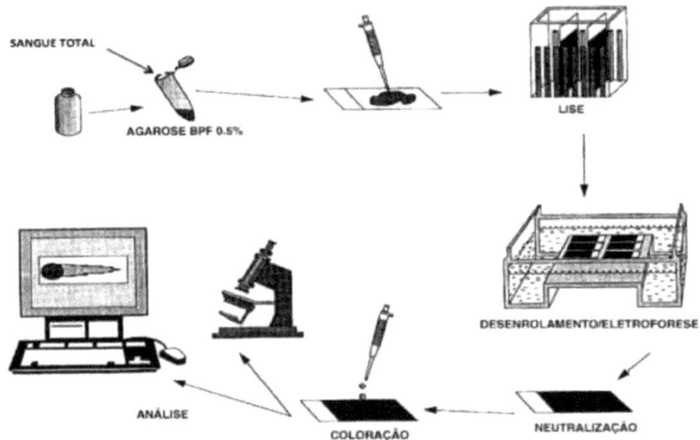

Figure 4: Summary of the comet assay stages. Source: adapted from DFT/INCQS/FIOCRUZ.

3.5 Biochemical evaluation of offspring whole blood.

Biochemical parameters were assessed using BIOCLIN (2012) semi-automated reagent kits, following the protocols available for glucose (Plasma - K082), triglycerides (Plasma - K117), total cholesterol (Plasma - K083), LDL (Plasma - K088), total protein (Serum - K031), albumin (Serum - K040), ALT (Plasma - K034), AST (Plasma - K035), total and ionized calcium (Plasma - K007).

3.6 Biochemical evaluation of milk

3.6.1 Triglycerides

Milk samples were taken on the 14th day of lactation. To do this, the mothers were separated from their offspring two hours before milking by hand (BONOMO *et al.*, 2005). They received subcutaneous oxytocin (1 mL; 5 IU) 15 minutes beforehand. Then, under anesthesia with pentobarbital (160 mg/Kg) (adapted from AIUB *et al.,* 2011), they were milked, each providing approximately 0.5 to 1.5 mL of milk volume. The samples were frozen at -20°C for later analysis. Triglycerides were measured in milk samples diluted in distilled water (1:25) by colorimetric assay using a commercial BIOCLIN kit (SANTOS- SILVA *et al.*, 2011). After milking, the rats were subjected to cardiac puncture and sacrificed.

3.7 Statistical analysis

For all tests, the T-STUDENT test was applied, comparing the treated groups to the control group. Differences were considered statistically significant when $p < 0.05$.

4. RESULTS

4.1 Toxicological evaluation in prokaryotes

4.1.1 Bacterial reverse mutation induction (Salmonella/microsome/Ames test)

In the mutagenicity test, using *Salmonella enterica* serovar Typhimurium strains TA97, TA98, TA100, TA102, TA104 and TA1535 (table 4), in the presence and absence of exogenous metabolization, sorbitol showed no mutagenicity (I.M. ≥ 2) for any of the strains and concentrations used, in the range of 0 to 4000 µg/plate. There was no cytotoxic response in the strains used, but a dose dependency in strains TA97, TA98 and TA102, in the presence of S9.

Table 4 - Mutagenicity test with *S. enterica* serovar Typhimurium strains TA97, TA98, TA100, TA102 and TA1535, in the presence and absence of S9 mix, incubated (72 h., at 37°C) with sorbitol 0; 0.4; 4; 40; 400 and 4000 µg/plate.

Cepa	µg/plate	- S9			+ S9		
		I.M.	Rev. ± D.P.	Under. %	I.M.	Rev. ± D.P.	Under. %
TA97	0	1,1	82,3 ± 12,1	100,0	1,0	225,0 ± 8,5	100,0
	0,4	0,7	51,5 ± 19,1	100,0	1,4	313,0 ± 24,9	100,0
	4	0,8	58,7 ± 15,6	100,0	0,7	165,0 ± 5,7	100,0
	40	0,9	67,5 ± 16,3	100,0	0,6	136,0 ± 5,7	100,0
	400	1.1	82,3 ± 17,2	100,0	0,6	135,0 ± 25,4	100,0
	4000	1,2	86,5 ± 2,1	100,0	0,6	134,5 ± 34,6	81,0
	5000	1,2	87,7 ± 5,9	100,0	0,6	131,5 ± 12,0	**64,3**
	C.P.	**4,3**	322,3 ± 23	92,1	**2,8**	624,3 ± 65,9	100,0
TA98	0	1,0	25,3 ± 3,1	100,0	1,0	43,0 ± 1,4	100,0
	0,4	1,0	23 ± 0	99,1	0,9	37,0 ± 4,2	89,1
	4	1,0	23,7 ± 2,3	86,7	0,9	38,0 ± 8,0	86,1
	40	1,0	25,3 ± 5,1	83,3	1,2	51,3 ± 2,3	86,1
	400	1,0	26,3 ± 8,5	75,9	1,2	51,3 ± 5,0	76,2
	4000	1,1	28,5 ± 4,9	74,4	1,7	71,3 ± 3,1	71,9
	5000	1,2	29,3 ± 7,6	72,5	1,8	78,7 ±3,1	**62,7**
	C.P.	**5,7**	144 ± 13	91,4	**7,1**	305,0 ± 1,4	95,1
TA100	0	1,0	116 ± 17	100,0	1,0	123,2 ± 11,0	100,0
	0,4	1,3	148 ± 30	100,0	1,1	136,0 ± 14,4	95,9
	4	1,1	128 ± 13,9	100,0	1,2	146,7 ± 44,5	95,0
	40	1,2	135 ± 20	100,0	1,0	119,3 ± 8,1	92,7
	400	1,5	170 ± 28	100,0	1,0	118,0 ± 6,0	91,9
	4000	1,3	153 ± 29	89,2	0,9	116,0 ± 10,6	90,4
	5000	1,3	149 ± 5,7	100,0	0,9	114,0 ± 5,7	88,6
	C.P.	**16,0**	1873 ±32	76,0	**5,8**	718,0 ± 19,8	98,3
TA102	0	1,0	439 ± 34	100,0	1,0	314,7 ± 12,1	100,0
	0,4	1,1	467 ± 60	98,7	1,1	344,0 ± 8,5	89,6
	4	1,0	458 ± 11	98,2	1,2	385,5 ± 7,8	87,5
	40	1,1	493 ± 32	94,9	1,3	411,3 ± 4,0	85,6

	400	1,1	485 ± 46	93,8	1,3	413,0 ± 7,1	84,3
	4000	1,1	493 ± 32	93.7	1,4	454,0 ± 9,8	81,2
	5000	1,4	578 ± 55	82,3	1,5	469,5 ± 9,2	**60,2**
	C.P.	**2,7**	1177 ±27	77,1	**4,4**	1393 ± 15,6	78,3
TA104	0	1,0	329 ± 28	100,0	1,0	661 ± 39,3	100,0
	0,4	1,1	349 ± 47	100,0	1,0	643 ± 47,6	86,02
	4	1,1	356 ± 17	100,0	1,0	668 ± 26,6	98,92
	40	1,1	359 ± 23	80,8	1,3	853 ± 12,7	91,4
	400	1,1	361 ± 46	78,9	1,3	852 ± 24,3	91,4
	4000	1,0	318 ± 32	85,8	1,3	853 ± 1,4	100,0
	5000	0,9	279 ± 16	77,6	1,3	880 ± 28,3	100,0
	C.P.	**2,3**	746 ± 58	70,6	**2,3**	1485 ± 21,6	100,0
TA1535	0	1,0	10 ± 2	100,0	1,0	13 ± 4,2	100,0
	0,4	1,0	10 ± 5	100,0	0,9	11 ± 4,2	100,0
	4	1,2	11,5 ± 0,7	100,0	0,8	10 ± 5,7	100,0
	40	1,3	13 ± 4	100,0	0,8	10 ± 3,4	100,0
	400	1,0	10 ± 3	100,0	0,8	10,7 ± 6,4	93,8
	4000	1,4	13,5 ± 0,7	100,0	0,9	12 ± 8,5	90,7
	5000	1,1	11 ± 1	100,0	0,8	10 ± 2,82	79,0
	C.P.	**2,4**	24,4 ± 51	**32,0**	**2,1**	27 ± 1,4	91,36

Results expressed as mean and standard deviation of triplicates. NC (Negative Control): water; PC with S9 mix (Positive Control with S9 mix): TA97, TA98, TA100, TA104 and TA1535 (Amino Anthracene 1.0 µg/plate); PC without S9 mix (Positive Control without S9 mix): TA97, TA98 and TA1535 (4-Nitroquinoline 1-oxide 1.0 µg/plate), TA102 and TA104 (Mitomycin C 0.5 µgZplate) and TA100 (Sodium Azide 1.0 µg/plate); I.M.: Mutagenicity index in relation to the negative control; S.D.: Standard Deviation; S.W.: Survival; Rev.: number of bacterial revertants; M.I. ≥ 2 (mutagenicity) and S.W. (cell survival) < 70% (cytotoxicity) in bold. As no result showed I.M. ≥ 2, with the exception of the positive control, statistics were not performed.

4.2 Maternal sorbitol intake during lactation

4.2.1 Treatment and monitoring of animals in vivaria

The rats in all groups (control: water; 0.00015 mg/g; 0.0015 mg/g and 0.15 mg/g), obtained from the central animal house at UFRJ, showed similar weight gain during pregnancy, with no statistically significant difference *($p < 0.05$)* (figure 5).

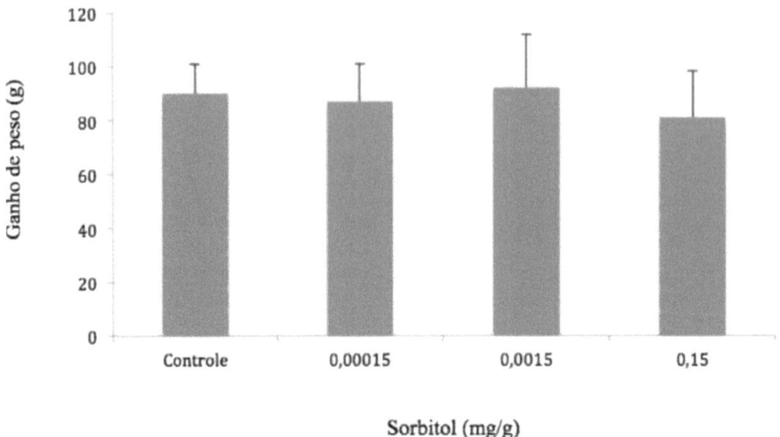

Figure 5 - Average weight gain of mothers at the end of pregnancy (control: water; 0.00015 mg/g; 0.0015 mg/g and 0.15 mg/g). The values represent the mean and standard deviation of 6 mothers per group. * p < 0,05.

The average number of births for each experimental group varied between 10 and 12. When comparing the results of the treated groups to the control (control: water; 0.00015 mg/g; 0.0015 mg/g and 0.15 mg/g), the group treated with 0.0015 mg/g sorbitol showed a statistically significant increase (20%) ($p < 0.05$), as shown in figure 6.

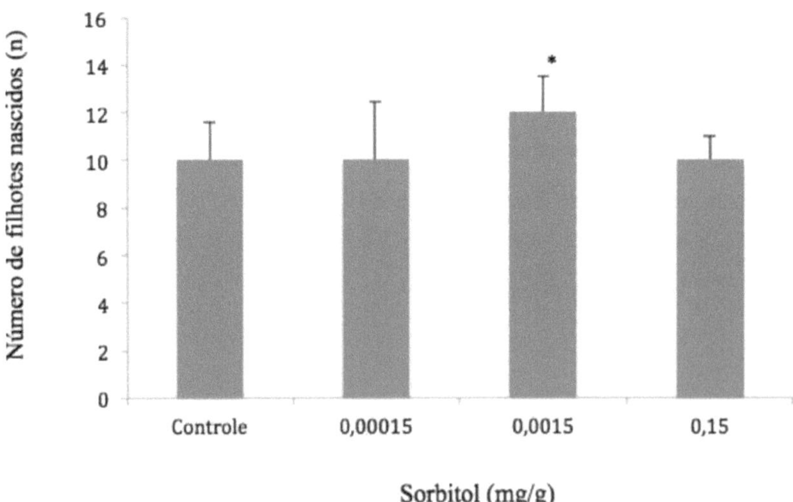

Figure 6 - Average number of pups born per experimental group (control: agıa; 0.00015 mg/g; 0.0015 mg/g and 0.15 mg/g). The values represent the mean and standard deviation of 6

chicks per group. * p < 0,05.

The averages for males (M) and females (F) of the offspring are shown in figure 7. They were homogeneously distributed for the majority of males. None of the treated groups (0.00015 mg/g; 0.0015 mg/g and 0.15 mg/g) showed any statistically significant difference ($p < 0.05$) compared to the control group (water).

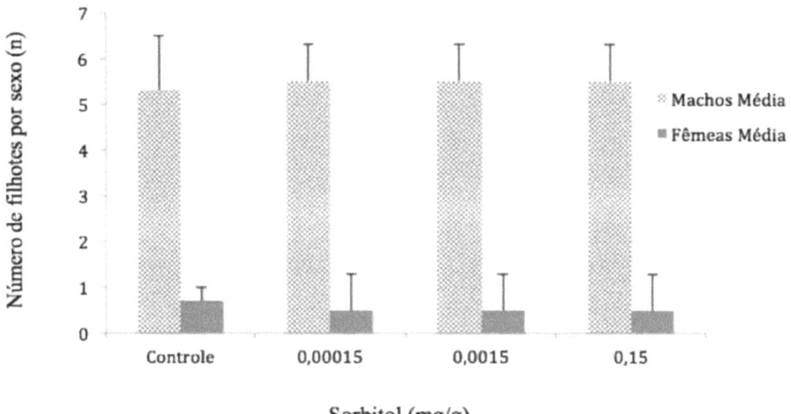

Figure 7 - Average number of males (M) and females (F) per experimental group (control: water; 0.00015 mg/g; 0.0015 mg/g and 0.15 mg/g). The values represent the mean and standard deviation of 6 pups per group. * $p < 0,05$.

4.3 Evaluation of weight, length, feed intake and water intake

At the end of the 14 days, there was a greater weight gain for the mothers who received sorbitol at concentrations of 0.00015 (113.3%) and 0.0015 (128%) mg/g, which were statistically significant ($p < 0.05$) compared to the control (figure 8).

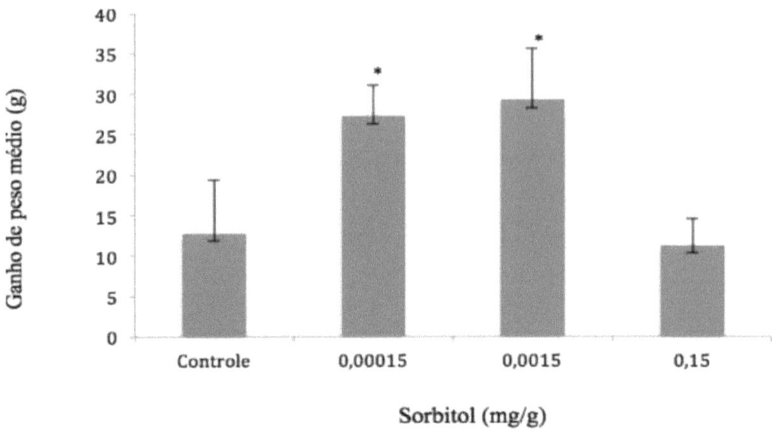

Figura 8 - Average weight gain of mothers at the end of 14 days of lactation (control: water; 0.00015 mg/g; 0.0015 mg/g and 0.15 mg/g). The values represent the mean and standard deviation of 6 mothers per group. * $p < 0,05$.

The pups of the mothers who received sorbitol at a concentration of 0.00015 mg/g gained more weight (28%) compared to the control and those who received sorbitol at a concentration of 0.15 mg/g lost weight (28%) compared to the control and these differences were statistically significant ($p < 0.05$) (figure 9).

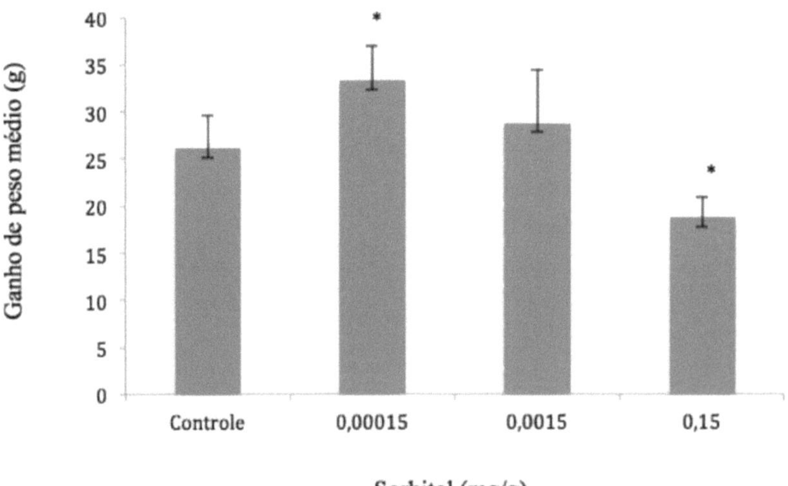

Figura 9 - Average weight gain of pups at the end of 14 days of lactation (control: water; 0.00015 mg/g; 0.0015 mg/g and 0.15 mg/g). The values represent the mean and standard deviation of 6 pups per group. *$p < 0,05$.

The offspring of all the groups (control: water; 0.00015 mg/g; 0.0015 mg/g and 0.15 mg/g) showed a similar profile in terms of average weight gain until the ninth day of lactation. From this day onwards, the 0.00015 mg/g and 0.0015 mg/g groups began to increase their weights in relation to the control, reaching 28% and 10%, respectively, at the end of the 14 days of lactation. The 0.15 mg/g group began to reduce its weight, also in relation to the control, reaching a 28% lower weight, also at the end of the 14 days of lactation. Only the 0.00015 mg/g and 0.15 mg/g groups showed statistically significant differences ($p < 0.05$) when compared to the control (water) at the end of 14 days of lactation, as shown in figure 10.

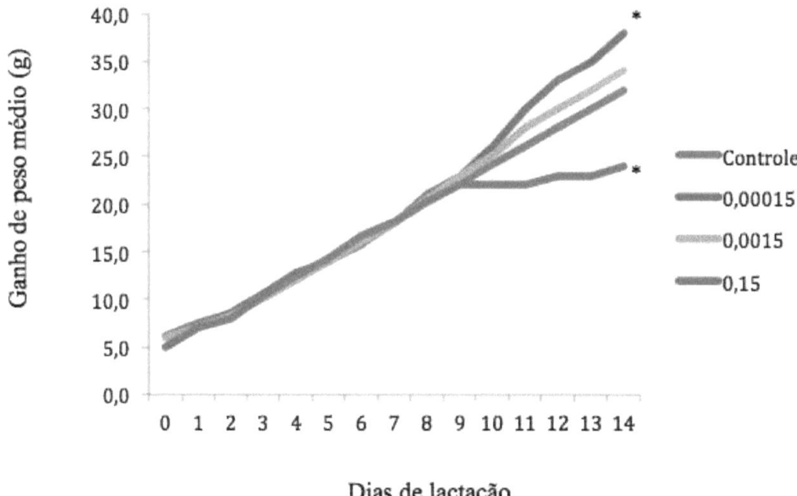

Figura 10 - Follow-up of the average weight gain of the pups in all the experimental groups (control: water; 0.00015 mg/g; 0.0015 mg/g and 0.15 mg/g) during the 14 days of lactation. The values represent the averages of 6 pups per experimental group. *$p < 0,05$.

The average length of the offspring was evaluated in centimeters during all 14 days of lactation and treatment. At the end of the 14 days, only the offspring of the mothers treated with the highest concentration (0.15 mg/g) showed a statistically significant reduction in length (9.5%) ($p < 0.05$) compared to the control (figure 11).

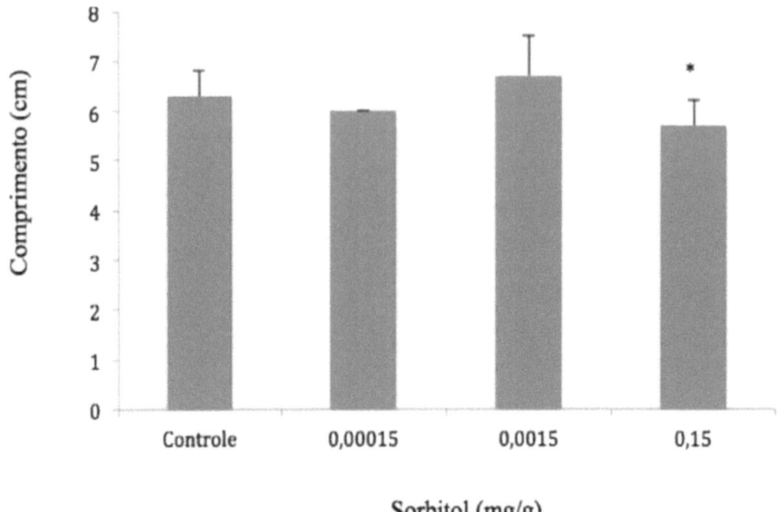

Figura 11 - Average length gain of pups at the end of 14 days of lactation (control: water; 0.00015 mg/g; 0.0015 mg/g and 0.15 mg/g). The values represent the mean and standard deviation of 6 pups per group. *$p < 0{,}05$.

The average feed consumption, as well as its kilocalorie equivalence, was evaluated during all 14 days of lactation in all groups (control: water; 0.00015 mg/g; 0.0015 mg/g and 0.15 mg/g) and showed a statistically significant reduction (33.3%) ($p < 0.05$) in the group of mothers that received the highest concentration, compared to the control (figure 12).

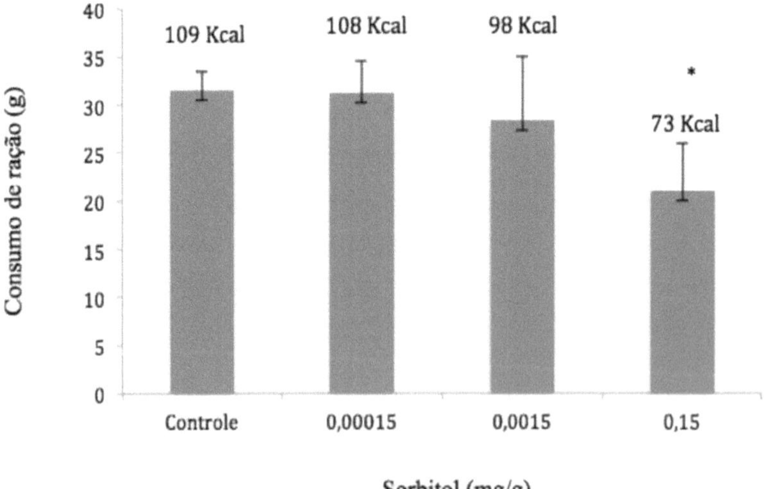

Figura 12 - Average feed consumption by mothers in all groups (control: water; 0.00015 mg/g; 0.0015 mg/g and 0.15 mg/g) during the 14 days of lactation. The values represent the mean and standard deviation of 6 mothers per group. *$p < 0,05$.

The treated groups (0.00015 mg/g; 0.0015 mg/g and 0.15 mg/g) showed no statistically significant differences compared to the control ($p < 0.05$), when we evaluated the average water intake of the mothers during the 14 days of lactation (figure 13).

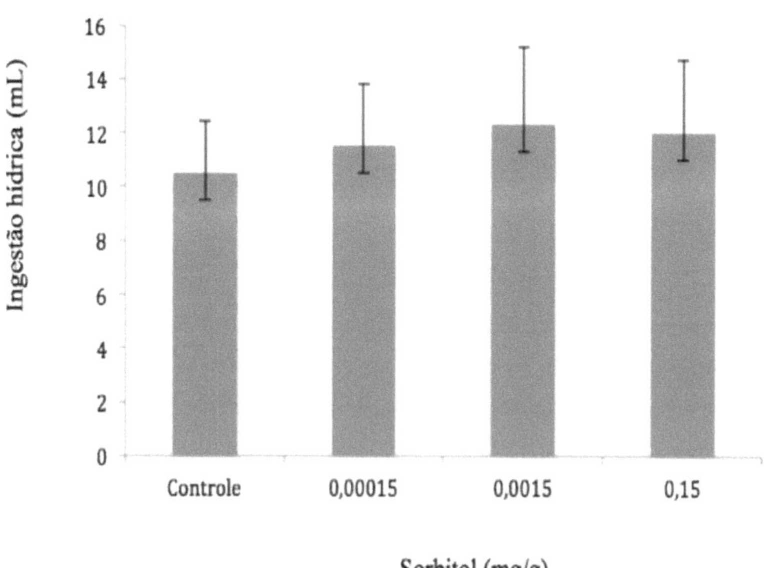

Figure 13 - Average water intake of mothers during the 14 days of lactation (0.00015 mg/g; 0.0015 mg/g and 0.15 mg/g). The values represent the mean and standard deviation of 6 mothers per group. *$p < 0,05$.

4.4 Biochemical evaluation of the offspring's whole blood

The blood *pools* of the suckled offspring in each mother rat treated with sorbitol 0.0015 mg/g and 0.15 mg/g showed a reduction in triglyceride levels (27%) and (40%), respectively. These were statistically significant ($p < 0.05$) compared to the control group (water) (figure 14).

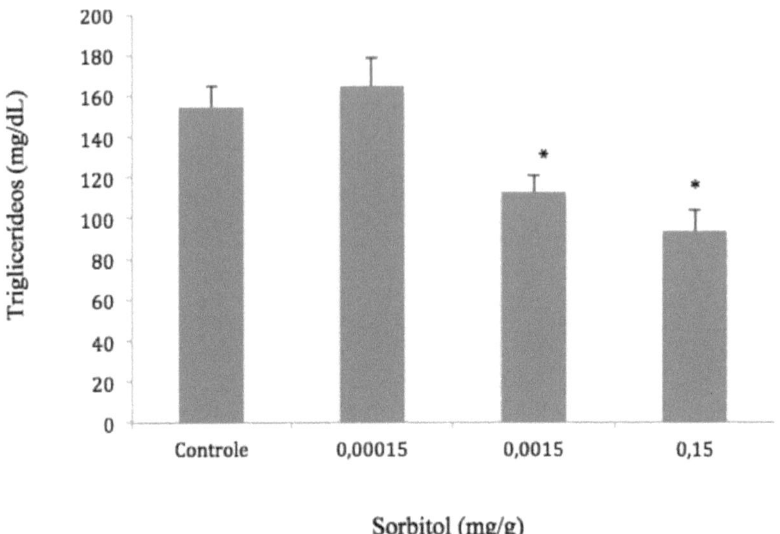

Figure 14 - Average triglyceride levels, in triplicate, in the blood of offspring from all groups (control: water; 0.00015 mg/g; 0.0015 mg/g and 0.15 mg/g), at the end of 14 days of lactation. The values represent the mean and standard deviation of 6 pups per group. *$p < 0,05$.

The level of total cholesterol in the blood of the offspring in the 0.00015 mg/g group increased by 42.7% compared to the control (water). This increase was statistically significant ($p < 0.05$), as shown in figure 15.

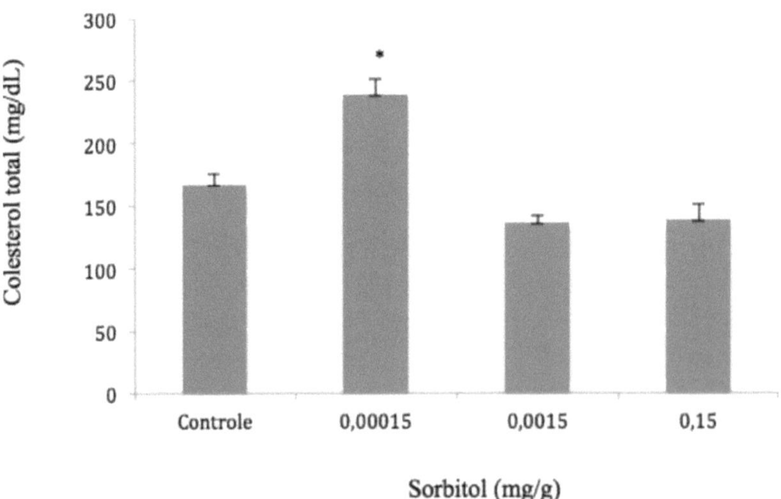

Figura 15 - Average total cholesterol levels, in triplicate, in the blood of offspring from all

groups (control: water; 0.00015 mg/g; 0.0015 mg/g and 0.15 mg/g), at the end of 14 days of lactation. The values represent the mean and standard deviation of 6 pups per group. *$p <$ 0,05.

The average blood glucose in the offspring of the 0.15 mg/g sorbitol group showed a statistically significant 20% reduction ($p < 0.05$) compared to the control (water) (figure 16).

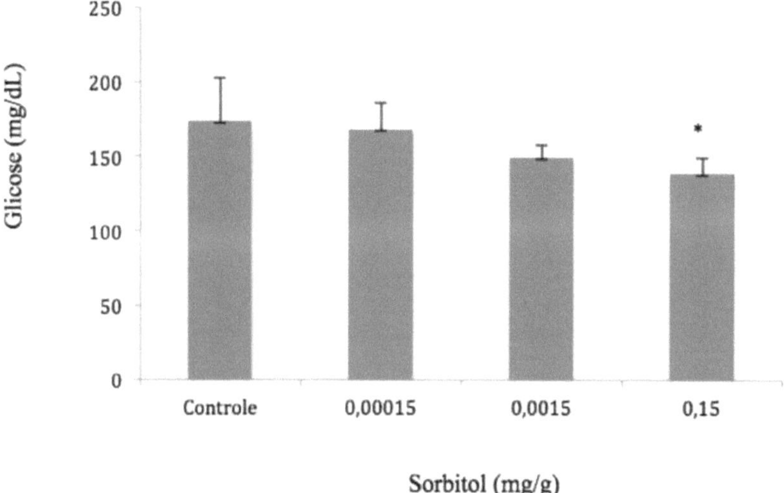

Figura 16 - Average glucose levels, in triplicate, in the blood of offspring from all groups (control: water; 0.00015 mg/g; 0.0015 mg/g and 0.15 mg/g), at the end of 14 days of lactation. The values represent the mean and standard deviation of 6 pups per group. *$p <$ 0,05.

The total visceral proteins of all the treated groups (0.00015 mg/g; 0.0015 mg/g and 0.15 mg/g) showed a statistically significant reduction ($p < 0.05$), 30.4%; 38.7% and 64.1%, respectively, when compared to the control group (water) (figure 17).

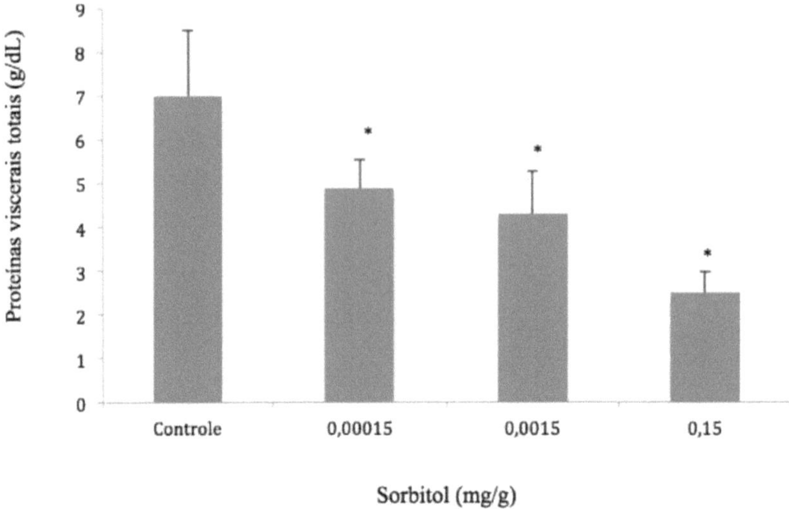

Figura 17 - Average dosage of total visceral proteins, in triplicate, in the blood of offspring from all groups (control: water; 0.00015 mg/g; 0.0015 mg/g and 0.15 mg/g), at the end of 14 days of lactation. The values represent the mean and standard deviation of 6 pups per group. ****$p < 0,05$*.**

The average albumin dosages, in triplicate, indicated a statistically significant reduction ($p < 0.05$) in the two highest concentrations (0.0015 mg/g and 0.15 mg/g), 17.3% and 33.2%, respectively (figure 18).

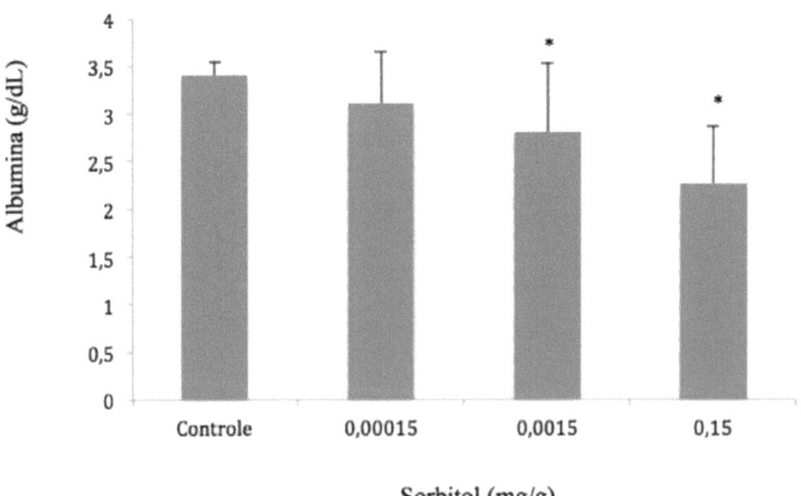

Figura 18 - Average albumin dosage, in triplicate, in the blood of the offspring of all groups (control: water; 0.00015 mg/g; 0.0015 mg/g and 0.15 mg/g), at the end of 14 days of lactation. The values represent the mean and standard deviation of 6 pups per group. *$p < 0,05$.

The average dosages of total calcium, in triplicate, indicated a statistically significant reduction ($p < 0.05$), in all groups (0.00015 mg/g; 0.0015 mg/g and 0.15 mg/g), 43.8%; 43.8% and 62.5%, respectively, in relation to the control group (water) (figure 19).

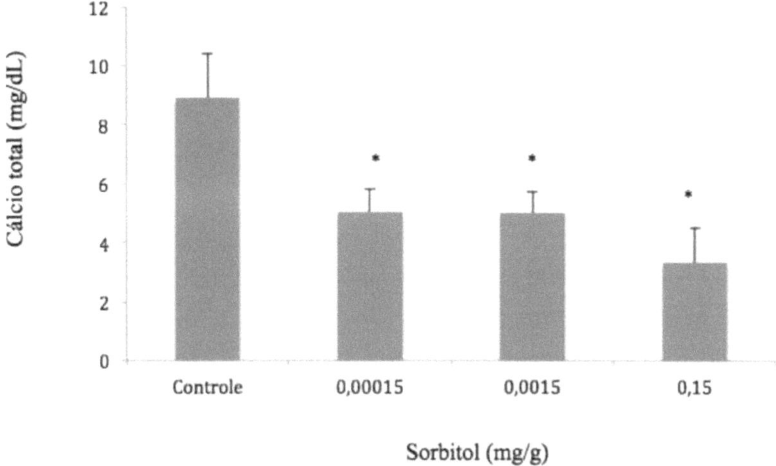

Figura 19 - Average total calcium levels, in triplicate, in the blood of offspring from all groups (control: water; 0.00015 mg/g; 0.0015 mg/g and 0.15 mg/g), at the end of 14 days of lactation. The values represent the mean and standard deviation of 6 pups per group. *p < 0,05.

After analysis of total calcium, ionized calcium was calculated. It corresponded to total calcium, with lower levels (40.5%, 38% and 54.4%, respectively) in the treated groups (0.00015 mg/g, 0.0015 mg/g and 0.15 mg/g) compared to the control group (water). All showed statistically significant differences ($p < 0.05$), as shown in figure 20.

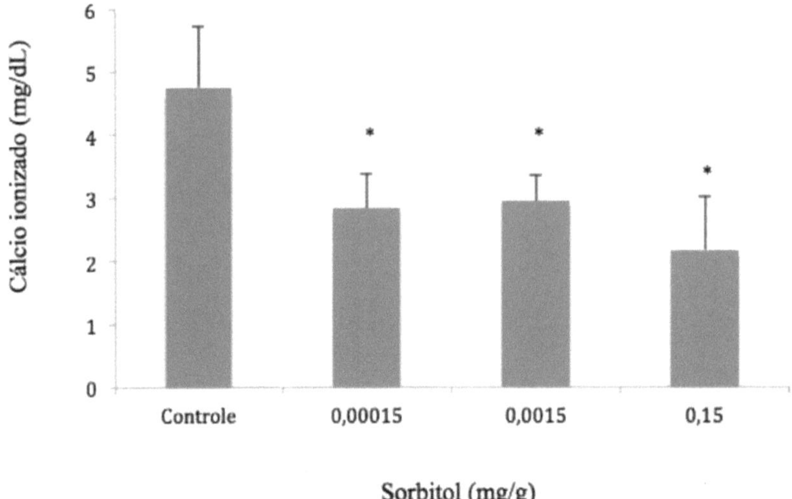

Figura 20 - Average dosage of ionized calcium, in triplicate, in the blood of the offspring of all groups (control: water; 0.00015 mg/g; 0.0015 mg/g and 0.15 mg/g), at the end of 14 days of lactation. The values represent the mean and standard deviation of 6 pups per group. *p < 0,05.

LDL cholesterol levels, in triplicate, were 38.3%, 35.8% and 35% higher in all the treated groups (0.00015 mg/g, 0.0015 mg/g and 0.15 mg/g), respectively, compared to the control group and all indicated statistically significant differences compared to the control group ($p < 0.05$), as shown in figure 21.

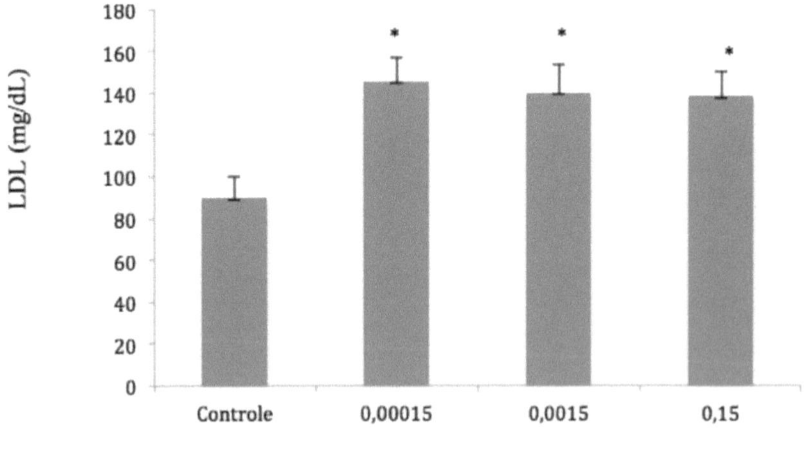

Figura 21 - Average LDL cholesterol fraction, in triplicate, in the blood of offspring from all groups (control: water; 0.00015 mg/g; 0.0015 mg/g and 0.15 mg/g), at the end of 14 days of lactation. The values represent the mean and standard deviation of 6 pups per group. *$p <$ 0,05.

Liver function was partially assessed by analyzing ALT levels, in triplicate, which indicated dose dependence between the treated groups (0.00015 mg/g; 0.0015 mg/g and 0.15 mg/g). However, it only showed statistically significant differences ($p < 0.05$) in the two highest concentrations (0.0015 mg/g and 0.15 mg/g), in which the increase was 15.9% and 159.6%, respectively, as shown in figure 22.

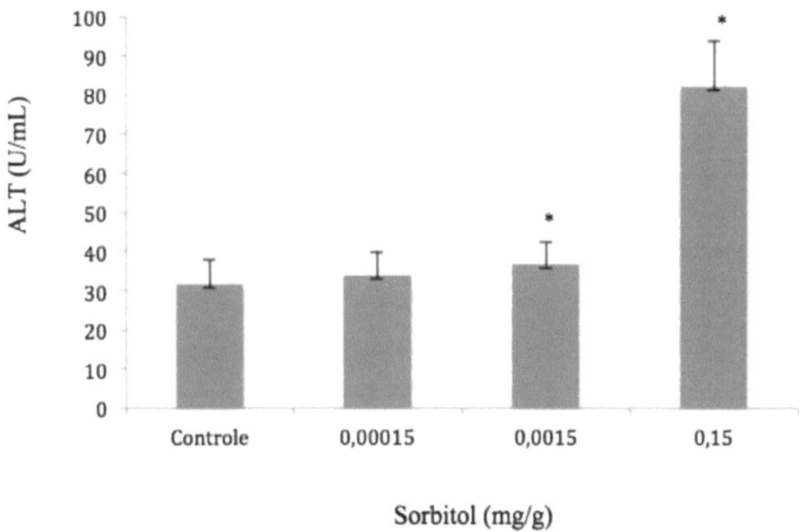

Figura 22 - Average ALT levels, in triplicate, in the blood of offspring from all groups (control: water; 0.00015 mg/g; 0.0015 mg/g and 0.15 mg/g), at the end of 14 days of lactation. The values represent the mean and standard deviation of 6 pups per group. *$p <$ 0,05.

The average AST dosages, in triplicate, indicated dose dependence at the highest levels, 69.2% and 475.3%, respectively, at the two highest concentrations (0.0015 mg/g and 0.15 mg/g), compared to the control. These showed statistically significant differences ($p < 0.05$), as shown in figure 23.

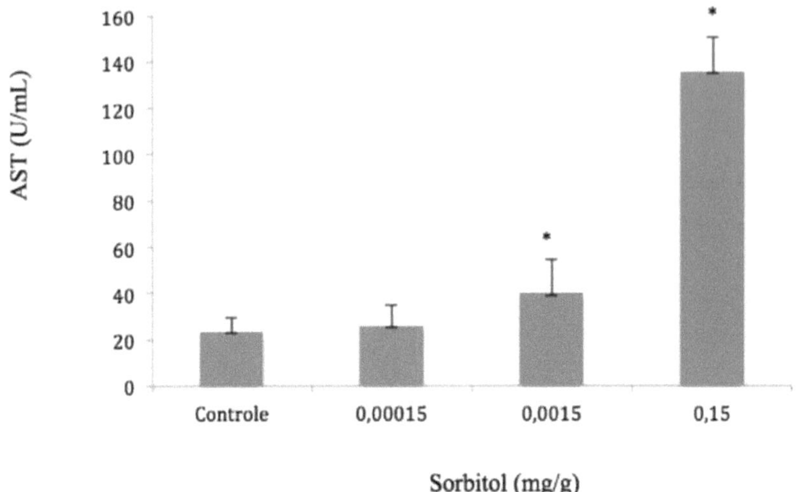

Figura 23 - Average AST levels, in triplicate, in the blood of offspring from all groups (control: water; 0.00015 mg/g; 0.0015 mg/g and 0.15 mg/g), at the end of 14 days of lactation. The values represent the mean and standard deviation of 6 pups per group. *p < 0,05.

4.5 Biochemical evaluation of milk from treated mothers

The mothers who received the lowest concentrations of sorbitol (0.00015 mg/g and 0.0015 mg/g) showed an increase in the amount of triglycerides in the milk, 62% and 3.8% respectively. These were statistically significant ($p < 0.05$) when compared to the control (water) (figure 24).

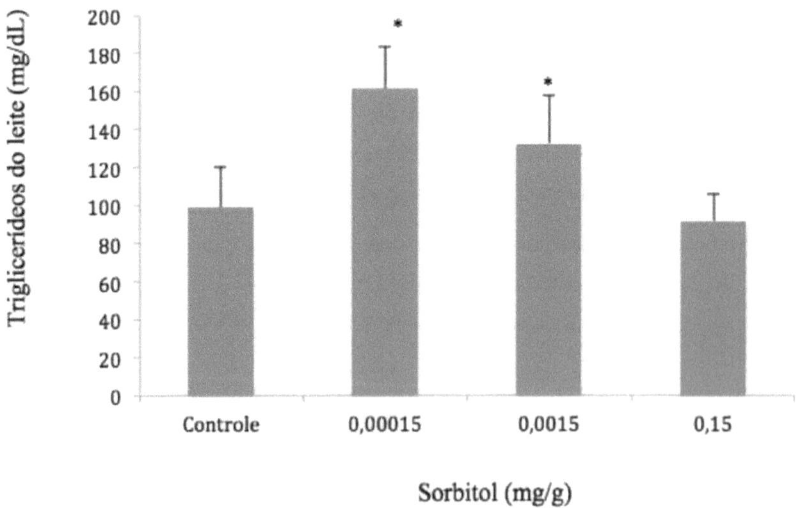

Figure 24 - Average dosage of triglycerides, in triplicate, in the milk of mothers in all groups

(control: water; 0.00015 mg/g; 0.0015 mg/g and 0.15 mg/g), at the end of 14 days of lactation. The values represent the mean and standard deviation of 6 mothers per group. *$p < 0,05$.

4.6 *In vivo* micronucleus and comet tests on mammalian cells

4.6.1 Micronucleus in hepatocytes

The offspring group (0.00015 mg/g) showed an increased number of micronucleated hepatocytes and apoptosis. The offspring of mothers treated with the highest concentration (0.15 mg/g) showed no increase in micronucleated cells. This group showed an increase in dividing cells, necrosis and apoptosis. All of the above results show statistically significant differences compared to the control ($p < 0.05$), as shown in Table 5.

Table 5 - Cytotoxic evaluation of sorbitol in primary hepatocyte culture of offspring

	CONTROL		0,00015		0,0015		0,15	
	M	DP	M	DP	M	DP	M	DP
MN	242 (24%)	30,6	**349** (35%)	46,5	**325** (32,5%)	38,3	245 (24,5%)	34,3
DC	274 (27%)	50,5	281 (28%)	48,3	**286** (28,6%)	44	**290** (29%)	21,5
NC	29 (3%)	7,8	28 (2,8%)	4,1	28 (2,8%)	2,7	**50** (5%)	6,5
APT	0,2 (0,02%)	0,4	**1,8** (0,2%)	0,7	1 (0,1%)	0,8	**2** (0,2%)	1,2

Results expressed as mean and standard deviation of quintuplicate. Control: water; M: mean; SD: standard deviation; MN: micronucleus; DC: cell division; NC: necrosis; APT: apoptosis: Standard Deviation; MN: micronucleus; DC: cell division; NC: necrosis; APT: apoptosis. Results that showed a statistically significant difference ($p < 0.05$) compared to the control are in bold.

4.6.2 Bone marrow micronucleus

In relation to the bone marrow micronucleus assay, all the treated groups showed statistically significant differences ($p < 0.05$) for all the parameters: micronucleus (MN), cell division (DC), necrosis (NC), apoptosis (APT), orthochromatic (Orto), polychromatic (Poli), micronucleated polychromatic (Poli MN) and the ratio between polychromatic and orthochromatic. The decreased number of normal polychromatic erythrocytes, increased number of micronuclei, decreased number of dividing cells and increased number of necrotic cells compared to the control are shown in Table 6.

Table 6 - Cytotoxic evaluation of sorbitol in bone marrow of offspring

CONTROL			0,00015		0,0015		0,15	
	AVERAGE	DP	AVERAGE	DP	AVERAGE	DP	AVERAGE	DP
MN	38 (10%)	4,0	**45** (11%)	2,1	**43** (11%)	3,1	**55** (14%)	3
DC	145 (36%)	16,6	**116** (29%)	7,2	**115** (29%)	1,9	**105** (26%)	6
NC	17 (4%)	2,2	**41** (10%)	6,7	**39** (10%)	10,5	**50** (12%)	5

APT	0 (0%)	0	**0,2** (0%)	0,2	**0,3** (0,1%)	0,3	**0,3** (0,1%)	0,3
Ortho	194 (48%)	13,9	**363** (91%)	3,1	**365** (91%)	4,1	**368** (92%)	4
Poli	206 (52%)	13,9	**39** (10%)	2,4	**34** (9%)	4,1	**32** (8%)	4
Poli MN	13 (3%)	4,3	**28** (7%)	1,6	**27** (7%)	2,9	**24** (6%)	5
Poli/Orto	1 (107%)	0,2	**0,1** (11%)	0	**0,1** (9%)	0	**0,1** (1%)	0

Results expressed as mean and standard deviation of quintuplicate. Control: water; SD: standard deviation; MN: micronucleus; DC: cell division; NC: necrosis; APT: apoptosis: SD: standard deviation; MN: micronucleus; DC: cell division; NC: necrosis; APT: apoptosis; Poli: polychromatic; Ortho: orthochromatic. Results that showed a statistically significant difference *($p < 0.05$)* compared to the control are in bold.

4.6.3 Comet

Taking into account the level of arbitrary units of the comet test, we identified an increase in dose-dependent genotoxicity. The means of all the treated groups showed a significant difference compared to the control ($p < 0.05$), as shown in Table 7.

Table 7 - Genotoxic evaluation of sorbitol in whole blood

	U.A.T	AVERAGE	DP	ERROR P	VARIANCE	TEST F	TEST T
	10,7						
	16,8						
C	14	14,36	2,74	1,22	7,49	-	-
	13						
	17,3						
	26						
	37,3						
0,00015	30,8	**32,26**	5,91	2,65	34,98	0,165	0,0001383
	39,5						
	27,7						
	62						
	77,3						
0,0015	64,3	**66,4**	6,18	2,76	38,19	0,144	0,00000007
	64,7						
	63,7						
	87,2						
	73,7						
0,15	79,2	**79,96**	7,1	3,16	50,06	0,093	0,00000003
	87,2						
	72,5						

Results expressed as mean and standard deviation of quintuplicate. C: control (water); SD: Standard Deviation; P: standard error; T: T-STUDENT test. Results that showed a statistically significant difference *($p < 0.05$)* compared to the control were highlighted in bold.

5. Discussion

The initial results of the mutagenicity test with strains of *Salmonella enterica* serovar Typhimurium made it possible to work with much lower concentrations of sorbitol when compared to the study by FUJITA & SASAKI (1986), and to expand the data on mutagenicity in different strains (TA98, TA100, TA104 and TA1535), meeting the requirements of the OECD (MARON & AMES, 1983; OECD 471, 1997; MORTELMANS & ZEIGER, 2000). None of the concentrations showed mutagenic capacity, however, the number of revertants varied in a dose-dependent manner, suggesting that other mechanisms, non-genotoxic and absent in bacterial cells, could be involved. The dose dependence in the absence of S9 may indicate a possible influence of P450 enzymes on the loss of this behavior (OECD 471, 1997; FDA, 2007). Survival of less than 70%, at the highest concentration in the presence of S9, is an expected result, so it did not affect the interpretation of the M.I. values. In an inversely proportional way, the Mutagenicity indices, in the presence of S9, decrease when the concentration of sorbitol per plate increases, indicating other possible metabolic influences. In the TA97 and TA100 strains, the M.I. decreased from the two lowest concentrations (0.4 and 4.0 µg/plate) to the three lowest (40; 400 and 4000 µg/plate). The specific nature of sorbitol, differences in metabolization and bioavailability may have influenced its effect on bacterial cells (OECD 471, 1997; FDA, 2007). Therefore, the results were negative under the test conditions, and the substance was not mutagenic for the species tested. This does not exempt sorbitol from a possible mutagenic and carcinogenic effect on mammalian cells. These facts justify the need for other complementary tests on blood, hematopoietic cells and hepatocytes.

The data from the follow-up in the vivarium suggests that sorbitol may be involved in adipogenesis. The groups were organized homogeneously in terms of the distribution of males and females, so that there was no influence of sexual dimorphism on day 14 (TROINA *et al.*, 2012). At the lowest concentration (0.00015 mg/g) they indicated greater weight gain in the mothers compared to the control group, reflected in a higher content of triglycerides in breast milk and increased weight gain in breastfed offspring. However, there was no correlation with plasma triglyceride levels, and there is a possibility that these triglycerides are being degraded into fatty acids and glycerol by the enzyme lipoprotein lipase and stored in adipogenic tissues. The latter parameters were not assessed in our study. The length of the offspring in this group showed no change compared to the control, suggesting an increase in Body Mass Index (BMI), which is associated with an increase in body fat and an altered lipid profile. According to NOVELLI *et al.* (2007), an increase in the Body Mass Index (BMI) of rats correlates well with an increase in biochemical parameters (lipid profile), corroborating our study, in which animals with an increased BMI showed an increase in Total Cholesterol (TC) and Low Density Lipoprotein (LDL), associated with possible cardiometabolic events (SOC BRAS CARDIOL, 2013). The preservation of normal levels of ALT, AST, albumin and changes in total visceral proteins alone indicate possible preservation of liver function. This is also indicated by increased synthesis of total cholesterol and LDL fraction.

The mothers that received sorbitol at a concentration of 0.0015 mg/g increased their milk weights and triglycerides, but without increasing their feed intake. This mechanism does not seem to be associated with appetite-disrupting pathways, only with an increase in the amount of sorbitol ingested and its influence on milk composition. This increase in milk resulted in a decrease in triglycerides in the plasma of the offspring, indicating no change in their weight or BMI. These changes suggest that sorbitol may be passing through the mother's milk, affecting important functions in metabolizing organs, such as the liver, and causing biochemical changes in the offspring, such as an increase in ALT, AST, a decrease in total visceral proteins and albumin, associated with an increase in LDL cholesterol fractions.

The intake of the highest concentration (0.15 mg/g) indicated a reduction in the feed intake of the mothers, weight and BMI of the breastfed offspring, associated with a reduction in length, which may indicate an increase in urinary excretion and a reduction in plasma calcium levels. These facts could stimulate a greater capacity of the intestine to absorb this mineral, however, in high concentrations, it has a proven laxative effect and may contribute to a reduction in its levels (CÀNDIDO & CAMPOS, 1996). The fact that the rats had a lower intake of dog food also corroborates the reduction in blood glucose. All these changes did not indicate a significant influence on milk triglyceride levels. This may indicate a direct influence of sorbitol on the offspring, such as a reduction in plasma triglyceride levels, associated with possible toxicity and liver hypofunction, also indicated by an increase in ALT and AST levels, a decrease in total visceral proteins, albumin and increased LDL in plasma. Data from HUNTER *et al.* (1978) and WILLIAN (1989), not evaluated in our study, suggest possible important endocrine contributions to weight reduction. According to the authors, an increased intake of sorbitol could contribute to a predisposition to adrenal medulla tumors, which would be associated with an increase in adrenaline in the blood, a fact that could influence changes in the animals' body composition.

Comparing the treated groups, total cholesterol levels were very similar to LDL levels in the two highest concentrations, a fact that could favor cardiometabolic events (SOC BRAS CARDIOL, 2013). However, when we analyzed the LDL level of the lowest concentration, we noticed that it was similar to that of the other groups, in addition to the fact that it showed a much higher total cholesterol level compared to the control and other treated groups. This higher level of cholesterol in the lower concentration may reflect the greater presence of other fractions, such as HDL and VLDL, which does not indicate a healthy cardiovascular profile, since, for example, the HDL fraction did not reduce the LDL fraction, even though it may be present in greater quantity.

Several studies suggest that sorbitol, in certain quantities, has harmful effects on health, associated with increased diuresis, increased calcium excretion, hypophosphatemia, hyperoxalemia, diabetic neuropathy, laxative stimulation, among others (RODGERS *et al.*, 2009; CÂNDIDO & CAMPOS, 1996; ASNAGHI *et al.,* 2003; ISLAM & SAKAGUCHI, 2006). It is known that daily calcium intake below the recommended values and changes in calcemia are associated with higher BMI, fat percentage, visceral and subcutaneous adipose tissue, increased waist circumference and that these factors are associated with possible changes in biochemical, metabolic and endocrine parameters, metabolic and endocrine parameters, such as a reduction in 1,25-dihydroxycholecalciferol concentrations, which may result in less transfer of the mineral to adipogenic body compartments, reducing lipogenesis and insulin production (ZEMEL *et al.*, 2000, 2004, 2005; ZEMEL, 2003; ST-ONGE, 2005; HEANEY, 2003). According to NOBRE *et al.* (2011; 2012), calcium was important in reversing endocrine and metabolic alterations in models of metabolic programming due to early weaning, with the possibility of this mechanism being associated with vitamin D inhibition, which strengthens the idea of its participation in the aforementioned events.

Evidence from ELLER & REIMER (2010a, 2010b) and ZANOBINI (1979) showed changes in liver metabolism, with variations in liver enzyme concentrations, depending on the quality of protein and calcium ingested, as well as the direct influence of sorbitol. There is the possibility that they try to obtain energy through alternative pathways, such as gluconeogenesis, in which there is an increase in lactic acid in the bloodstream and a consequent reduction in free calcium concentrations, supposed parameters that we did not measure in our study.

These changes in blood concentrations of calcium may reflect on its bioavailability to cells, favoring such changes, as in the study by JACQMAIN *et al.* (2003), in which dietary habits were associated with the intake of amounts of calcium (< 600 mg; 600 - 1000 mg and > 1000 mg/day) in humans between 20 and 65 years of age, both sexes. There was a dose-dependent correlation in the reduction of adipogenesis, reduction of total cholesterol, LDL fraction and triglycerides in more than 400 individuals. This change in lipid profile is also evidenced in the work of MAJOR *et al.* (2008). The mechanism seems to involve 1,25 dihydroxycholecalciferol (calcitriol), since it can influence the bioavailability of calcium to important intracellular compartments, such as the pancreas and adipocytes. In the pancreas it can increase insulin secretion and in the adipocyte it can stimulate the transcription factor for fatty acid synthase and, consequently, lipogenesis, inhibiting lipolysis when the level of calcium in the blood is low. These mechanisms seem to be better controlled by dietary sources of calcium (ZEMEL, 2003; ST-ONGE, 2005). This greater influence of dietary sources of calcium may be due to their correspondence with good sources of protein, which have supposedly been linked to weight loss in rats (ELLER & REIMER, 2010a, 2010b). Similarly, HUTH *et al.* (2006) showed that, clinically, a calcium intake (500 - 1300 mg/day), associated with a low-calorie diet (500 Kcal/day), can decrease weight and fat percentage, compared to a control, especially when dietary choices are made instead of supplements. However, YANOVSKI *et al.* (2009) found no statistically significant differences when they subjected their patients to a randomized controlled clinical trial with 1500 mg/day supplementation for two years. Just as there are studies associating calcium with weight loss, there are studies with calcium supplementation that have no statistically significant association with a reduction in body weight (TROWMAN *et al.*, 2006; LOAN, 2009).

The results presented in the bone marrow micronucleus assay show a dose-dependent cytotoxicity associated with the consumption of sorbitol at all concentrations. Therefore, sorbitol may induce damage to erythroblasts of the *wistar* rat strain, resulting in a decrease in the number of dividing cells and an increase in necrotic cells. The latter show morphological changes that appear after cell death in living tissue. The progressive action of enzymes on lethally, irreversibly, progressively and degeneratively injured cells fails to maintain the integrity of the pyosmotic membrane, allowing its contents to leak out and potentially causing inflammation in adjacent tissues (KUMAR *et al.*, 2010).

The cytotoxicity of the bone marrow micronucleus test corroborates the micronucleus test in primary hepatocyte culture, in which all the treated groups showed at least one of the parameters evaluated (Micronucleus, Necrosis or Apoptosis) with statistically significant higher values, between 1 and 8% ($p < 0.05$), when compared to the control group. At the two lowest concentrations, where the animals with the greatest weight gain were found, we did not find cell necrosis; however, looking at the highest concentration, we can see that both necrosis and apoptosis differ significantly from the control group. Apoptosis is also a type of cell death, but it is programmed and controlled intracellularly, through the activation of enzymes that degrade nuclear DNA and cytoplasmic proteins, with an integral membrane and little morphological change, so that the phagocyte recognizes it. As a result, it is quickly eliminated, with no time for extravasation of the contents, followed by inflammation (KUMAR *et al.*, 2010). In our study, we evaluated an induced process of apoptosis, since the cell does not reach its maximum rate of division.

According to the Ministry of Health (2010), sorbitol is classified as being used with caution during lactation, as there is not enough information to determine its passage through breast milk, a method included in our perspectives. The pathway of sorbitol in our project involves passage through the digestive tract, blood and liver metabolism. There is also the possibility of a free part reaching the cells of the mammary gland through the plasma, being metabolized or not and passing directly or indirectly through breast milk, generating possible complications in the metabolism of breastfed offspring.

6. CONCLUSIONS

- The intake of sorbitol by lactating *Wistar* rats at different concentrations (0.00015, 0.0015 mg/g and 0.15 mg/g) resulted in nutritional, biochemical and toxicological alterations in the breastfed offspring after 14 days of treatment.

- The intake of sorbitol 0.00015 mg/g by lactating *wistar* rats led to weight gain in the mothers and breastfed offspring, an increase in total cholesterol and LDL fraction, a reduction in total visceral proteins, total and ionized calcium in the offspring, as well as an increase in triglycerides in the milk of the lactating rats after 14 days of treatment.

- The intake of sorbitol 0.0015 mg/g by lactating *wistar* rats caused weight gain in the mothers, a reduction in triglycerides, an increase in LDL, a reduction in total and ionized calcium levels, an increase in ALT and AST, a reduction in total visceral proteins and albumin in the blood of the offspring and an increase in triglyceride levels in the milk of the lactating rats after 14 days of treatment.

- The intake of sorbitol 0.15 mg/g by lactating *wistar* rats led to a reduction in the mother's feed intake, a reduction in the weight and length of the breastfed offspring, a reduction in blood glucose, triglycerides, total visceral proteins, albumin, total and ionized calcium and an increase in LDL, ALT and AST after 14 days of treatment.

- Sorbitol was able to alter the composition of breast milk, increasing the amount of triglycerides, as a result of the decrease in concentrations offered to lactating women.

- The highest concentration of sorbitol (0.15 mg/g) appears to be cytotoxic and genotoxic to breastfed offspring, based on the whole blood comet and micronucleus tests, both in bone marrow and hepatocytes, resulting in a reduction in feed consumption and alterations in the nutritional, biochemical and toxicological profiles of breastfed offspring.

- None of the sorbitol concentrations, between 0.4 and 4000 µg/plate, was mutagenic in the *Samonella/microsome* assay, for strains TA97, TA98, TA100, TA102, TA104 and TA1535, in the presence and absence of metabolization.

7. REFERENCES

AIUB CAF, GADERMAIER G, OLIVEIRA I, FELZENSZWALB I, FERREIRA F, PINTO LFR, ECKL P. N-Nitrosodiethylamine genotoxicity in primary rat hepatocytes: Effects of cytochrome P450 induction by Phenobarbital. **Toxicol**, v. 10, p. 2340 - 2348, 2011.

AIUB, C. A.; PINTO, L. F.; FELZENSZWALB, I. Standardization of conditions for the metabolic activation of N-nitrosodiethylamine in mutagenicity tests. **Genetics and Molecular Research**, v. 3, n. 2, p. 264-272, 2004.

NATIONAL HEALTH SURVEILLANCE AGENCY. Breastfeeding and the use of medicines and other substances, ed. 2, 2010b.

NATIONAL HEALTH SURVEILLANCE AGENCY. Law 9782 of January 26, 1999.

NATIONAL HEALTH SURVEILLANCE AGENCY. Ordinance 540 of October 27, 1997.

NATIONAL HEALTH SURVEILLANCE AGENCY. RDC No. 18, of March 24, 2008.

NATIONAL HEALTH SURVEILLANCE AGENCY. RDC No. 27, of August 6, 2010a.

AMERICAN DIETETIC ASSOCIATION. Position of the American Dietetic Association: use of nutritive and nonnutritive sweeteners. **J Am Diet Assoc**. v. 104, n. 2, p. 255-275, 2004.

ASNAGHI V, GERHARDINGER C, HOEHN T, ADEBOJE A, LORENZI M. A role for polyol pathway in the early neuroretinal apoptosis and glial changes induced by diabetes in the rat. **Diabetes**, v. 52, p. 506-511, feb. 2003.

BANTLE, JP. Clinical aspects of sucrose and fructose metabolism. In: KRETCHMER, Norman: HOLLENBECK, Clarie B. (Ed.). **Sugars and Sweeteners**. Boca Raton: CRC Press, p. 51-62. 1991.

BARREIROS RC, BOSSOLAN G, TRINDADE CEP. Fructose in humans: metabolic effects, clinical utilization, and associated inherent errors. **Rev. Nutr**, v. 18, n. 3, p. 377-389, May/June, 2005.

BONOMO IT, LISBOA PC, PASSOS MC, PAZOS-MOURA CC, REIS AM, MOURA EG. Prolactin inhibition in lactating rats changes leptin transfer through the milk. **Hormone Metabolic Research**. v. 37, p. 220-225, 2005.

BOSCO A, LERARIO AC, SORIANO D, DOS SANTOS RF, MASSOTE P, GALVAO D, FRANCO ACHM, PURISCH S, FERREIRA A R. Retinopatia diabetica. **Arq Bras Endocrinol Metab**, v. 49, n. 2, p. 217-227, 2005.

BRUGNERA VF, BARUFFI R, PANATTO E. Use of sweeteners during pregnancy and lactation. **Revista Eletrônica Multidisciplinar Pindorama**, n. 2, jun., 2012.

CÂNDIDO LMB, CAMPOS AM. Sweeteners. In: **Alimentos para fins especiais: dietéticos**. Sao Paulo: Varela; 1996. p. 115-258.

CARMO EH, BARRETO ML, JUNIOR JBS. Changes in the morbidity and mortality patterns of the Brazilian population: the challenges for a new century. **Epidemiologia e Serviços de Saùde**, v. 12, n. 2, p. 63-75, apr/jun. 2003.

CASTRO AGP; FRANCO LJ. Characterization of the consumption of alternative sweeteners and dietetic products by diabetic individuals. **Arq Bras Endocrinol Metab**, v. 46 n. 3. p. 280-287, 2002.

CEDERROTH CR, NEF S. Fetal programming of adult glucose homeostasis in mice. **Plos one**, v. 4, n.9, p. 1-7, sept, 2009.

CHAVES GV, DE SOUZA DS, PEREIRA SE, SABOYA CJ, PERES WAF. Association between non-alcoholic fatty liver disease and liver function/injury markers with metabolic syndrome components in class III obese individuals. **Rev Assoc Med Bras**, v. 58, n. 3, p. 288-293, 2012.

CODEX ALIMENTARIUS. International Foods Standards. **Food and Agriculture Organization of the United Nations**, 2012.

COLLINS AR. The comet assay for DNA damage and repair: principles, applications, and limitations. **Mol Biotechnol**, v. 26, n. 3, p. 249-61, mar., 2004.

DEIERLEIN AL, SIEGA-RIZ AM, ADAIR LS, HERRING AH. Effects of Pre-Pregnancy Body Mass Index and Gestational Weight. Gain on Infant Anthropometric Outcomes. **J Pediatr**, p. 1-6, 2010.

DRUZIAN JI, DOKI C, SCAMPARINI. Simultaneous determination of sugars and polyols by high performance liquid chromatography (HPLC-IR) in low calorie ice cream ("DIET"/"LIGHT"). Ciênc. Tecnol. Aliment., v. 25, n. 2, p. 279-284, 2005.

ELLER LK, REIMER RA. Dairy Protein Attenuates Weight Gain in Obese Rats Better Than Whey or Casein Alone. **Obesity**, v. 18, p. 704-711, 2010a.

ELLER LK, REMER RA. A High Calcium, Skim Milk Powder Diet Results in a Lower Fat Mass in Male, Energy-Restricted, Obese Rats More Than a Low Calcium, Casein, or Soy Protein Diet. **J Nutr**, v. 140, p. 1234-1241, may, 2010b.

FIGUEIREDO MS; MOURA EG, LISBOA PC, ANDRADE TA, TREVENZOLI IH, OLIVEIRA E, BOAVENTURA GT, PASSOS MCF. Flaxseed supplementation of rats during lactation changes the adiposity and glucose homeostasis of their offspring. **Life Sci**. v. 85, p. 365-371, 2009.

FOOD AND DRUG ADMINISTRATION. Food fot human consumption. **Food and drugs.** v. 3.

Apr, 2012.

FOOD AND DRUG ADMINISTRATION. Toxicological Principles for the Safety Assessment of Food Ingredients. Chapter IV.C.1.a. **Bacterial Reverse Mutation Test**. jul, 2007.

FUJITA H, SASAKI M. Mutagenicity test of food additives with *Salmonella typhimurium* TA97 and TA102. **Kenkyu Nenpo Tokyo Toritsu Eisei Kenkyusho**, v. 37, p. 447-452, 1986.

HALLFRISCH J. Metabolic effects of dietary fructose. **FASEB J**. v. 4, n. 9, p.2652-2660, 1990.

HEANEY, R.P. Normalizing calcium intake: projected population effects for body weight. **J Nutr**, v. 133, p. 268-270, 2003.

HUNTER B, COLLEY J, STREET A, HEYWOOD R, PRENTICE D, MAGNUSSON G. Xylitol tumorigenicity and toxicity study in long-term dietary administration to rats. Huntingdon Research Center. World Health Organization. **JECFA**, 1978.

HUTH PJ, DIRIENZO DB, MILLER GD. Major Scientific Advances with Dairy Foods in Nutrition and Health. **J Dairy Sci**, v. 89, p. 1207-1221, 2006.

BRAZILIAN Institute of Geography and STATISTICS. Family budget survey. Analysis of Personal Food Consumption in Brazil. 2009.

NATIONAL INSTITUTE FOR HEALTH QUALITY CONTROL. Department of Pharmacology and Toxicology. FiOCRUZ. Comet assay protocol. 2009.

INSTITUTE OF MEDICINE. Weight gain during pregnancy: reexamining the guidelines, may, 2009.

ISLAM MS, SAKAGUCHI E. Sorbitol-based osmotic diarrhea: possible causes and mechanism of prevention investigated in rats. **World J Gastroenterol**, v. 12, n. 47, p. 76357641, dec. 2006.

JACQMAIN M, DOUCET E, DESPRÉS JP, BOUCHARD C, TREMBLY A. Calcium intake, body composition, and lipoprotein-lipid concentrations in adults. **Am J Clin Nutr**, v. 77, p. 1448-52, 2003.

JAUNIAUX E, HEMPSTOCK, TENG C, BATTAGLIA FC, BURTON GJ. Polyol concentrations in the fluid compartments of the human conceptus during the first trimester of pregnancy : maintenance of redox potential in a low oxygen environment. **J Clin Endocrinol Metab**, v. 90, n. 2, p. 1171-1175, feb. 2005.

JOINT FAO/WHO EXPERT COMMITTEE ON FOOD ADDITIVES. **Food and Agriculture Organization of The United Nations**. Geneva, June 2012.

KHADER M, ECKL PM and BRESGEN N. Effects of aqueous extracts of medicinal plants on

MNNG-treated rat hepatocytes in primary cultures. **J. Ethnopharmacol**, v. 112, p. 199202, 2007.

KUMAR V, ABBAS AK, FAUSTO N, ASTER JC. Cellular responses to stress and toxic stimuli: adaptation, injury and death. **Robbins & Cotran pathology Pathological Basis of Disease**, ch. 1, p. 3-39, ed. 8, 2010.

LEE BA, ZUMBE A, STOREY D. Breath hydrogen after ingestion of the bulk sweeteners sorbitol, isomalt and sucrose in chocolate. **Brit J Nut**, v. 71, p. 731-737, 1994.

LEVY-COSTA RB, SICHIERI R, PONTES NS, MONTEIRO CA. Household food availability in Brazil: distribution and trends (1974-2003). **Rev. Saùde Pùblica**, v. 39, n. 4, p. 1-10, apr. 2005.

LOAN MV. The Role of Dairy Foods and Dietary Calcium in Weight Management. **Journal of the American College of Nutrition**, v. 28, n. 1, p. 120S-129S, 2009.

MAJOR GC, CHAPUT JP, LEDOUX M, ST-PIERRE S, ANDERSON GH, ZEMEL MB. Tremblay A. Recent developments in calcium-related obesity research. **Obes Rev.** v. 9, p. 428-45, 2008.

MARON, D. M.; AMES, B. N. Revised methods for the Salmonella mutagenicity test. **Mutation Research**, v. 113, n. 3-4, p. 173-215, 1983.

MERCOSUR/GMC/RES. Criteria for determining additive functions and their maximum limits for all food categories. **Technical Regulation**, n. 52, 2008.

MOHN, G. R. Bacterial systems for carcinogenicity testing. **Mutation Research**, v. 87, n. 2, p. 191-210, 1981.

MORTELMANS K, ZEIGER, E. The Ames Salmonella/microsome mutagenicity assay. **Mutation Research**, v. 450, p. 29-60, 2000.

MOURA EG, LISBOA PC, PASSOS MCF. Neonatal programming of neuroimmunomodulation - role of adipocytokines and neuropeptides. **Neuroimmunomodulat**, v. 15, n. 3, p. 176-188, 2008.

MUIR JG, ROSE R, ROSELLA O, LIELS K, BARRETT JS, SHEPHERD SJ, GIBSON PR. Measurement of short-chain carbohydrates in common Australian vegetables and fruits by high-performance liquid chromatography (HPLC). **J. Agric. Food Chem**, v. 59, n. 2, p. 554565, 2009.

NATIONAL HEALTH AND NUTRITION EXAMINATION SURVEY. Data Documentation, Codebook, and Frequencies. Pregnancy Results. 2003-2004.

NOBRE, JL, LISBOA PC, SANTOS-SILVA AP, MANHÂES AC, NOGUEIRA-NETO JF ; CABANELAS A, PAZOS-MOURA CC, MOURA EG, OLIVEIRA E. Calcium supplementation reverses central adiposity, leptin, and insulin resistance in adult offspring programmed by neonatal nicotine exposure, **J Endocrinol**, v. 210, p. 349-49, 2011.

NOBRE, JL, LISBOA PC , LIMA NS, FRANCO JG, NOGUEIRA-NETO JF ; MOURA EG, OLIVEIRA E. Calcium supplementation prevents obesity, hyperleptinaemia and hyperglycaemia in adult rats programmed by early weaning. **Br J Nutr**. v. 107, n. 7, p. 979988, 2012.

NOVELLI ELB, DINIZ YS, GALHARDI CM, EBAID GMX, RODRIGUES HG, MANI F, FERNANDES AAH, CICOGNA AC, NOVELLI FILHO JLVB. **Laboratory Animals**, v. 41, p. 111-119, 2007.

OLIVEIRA PSM, FERREIRA VF, DE SOUZA MV. D-Mannitol in Organic Synthesis. **Quim Nova**, v. 32, n. 2, 2009.

ORGANIZATION FOR ECONOMIC CO-OPERATION AND DEVELOPMENT. OECD guideline for testing of chemicals: bacterial reverse mutation test. 1997. Available at: http://www.oecd.org. Accessed on: Mar. 2013.

ORGANIZATION FOR ECONOMIC CO-OPERATION AND DEVELOPMENT. OECD guideline for testing of chemicals: in vitro mammalian cell micronucleus test. 2010. Available at: http://www.oecd-ilibrary.org. Accessed on: Mar. 2013.

ORGANIZATION FOR ECONOMIC CO-OPERATION AND DEVELOPMENT. OECD guideline for testing of chemicals: mammalian erythrocyte micronucleus test. 1997. Available at: http://www.oecd-ilibrary.org. Accessed on: Mar. 2013.

PERES CM; CURI R. Como cultivar células. **Guanabara Koogan**. 2005.

PURCHASE, I. F. International Commission for Protection against Environmental Mutagens and Carcinogens. ICPEMC working paper 2/6. An appraisal of predictive tests for carcinogenicity. **Mutation Research**, v. 99, n. 1, p. 53-117, 1982.

RENWICK AG, MOLINARY SV. Sweet-taste receptors, low-energy sweeteners, glucose absorption and insulin release. **Br J Nutr**, p. 1-6, may, 2010.

ROCHA DS, NETTO MP, PRIORI SE, DE LIMA NMM, ROSADO LEFP, FRANSESCHINI SCC. Nutritional status and iron deficiency anemia in pregnant women: relationship with infant birth weight. **Revista de Nutriçâo.** Campinas, v. 4, n. 18, p. 481-489, jul/ago. 2005.

RODGERS A, BUNGANE N, ALLIE-HAMDULAY S, LEWANDOWSKI S, WEBBER D. Calciuria, oxaluria and phosphaturia after ingestion of glucose, xylitol and sorbitol in two population groups with different stone-risk profiles. **Urol Res**, v. 37, p. 121-125, 2009.

RONNBERG AK, NILSON K. Interventions during pregnancy to reduce excessive gestational weight gain: a systematic review assessing current clinical evidence using the Grading of

Recommendations, Assessment, Development and Evaluation (GRADE) system. **BJOG**, v. 117, n. 11, p. 1327-1334, oct., 2010.

SANTOS-SILVA AP, OLIVEIRA E, PINHEIRO CR, NUNES-FREITAS AL, ABREU-VILLAÇA Y, SANTANA AC, NASCIMENTO SABA CC, NOGUEIRA-NETO JF, REIS AM, MOURA EG, LISBOA PC. Effects of tobacco smoke exposure during lactation on nutritional and hormonal profiles in mothers and offspring. **Journal of Endocrinology**. v. 209, p. 75-84, 2011.

SAUNDERS C, PADILHA PC, LIMA HT, OLIVEIRA LM, QUEIROZ JA, THEME MLM. Literature review on recommendations for the use of sweeteners in pregnant women with diabetes mellitus. **FEMINA**. v. 38, n. 4, abr., 2010.

SHAFRIR E. Fructose/sucrose metabolism its physiological and pathological implications. In: KRETCHMER, Norman: HOLLENBECK, Clarie B. (Ed.). **Sugars and Sweeteners**. Boca Raton: CRC Press. p. 63-98, 1991.

BRAZILIAN SOCIETY OF CARDIOLOGY. First guideline on fat consumption and cardiovascular health. **Arq Bras Cardiol**. v. 100, n. 1, jan. 2013.

SOUZA AM, BEZERRA IM, CUNHA DB, SICHIERI R. Evaluation of food intake markers in the Brasilian surveillance system for chronic diseases - VIGITEL (2007-2009). **Rev Bras Epidemiol**. v. 14, n. 1, p. 44-52, 2011.

ST-ONGE MP. Dietary fats, teas, dairy, and nuts: potential functional foods for weight control? **Am J Clin Nutr**, v. 81, p. 7-15, 2005.

STULBACH TE, BENÎCIO MHA, ANDREAZZA R, KONO S. Determinants of excessive weight gain during pregnancy in a public low-risk prenatal service. **Rer Bras Epidemiol**, v. 10, n. 1, p. 99-108, 2007.

TORLONI MR, NAKAMURA MU, MEGALE A, SANCHEZ VHSS, MANO C, FUSARO AS, MATTAR R. The use of sweeteners in pregnancy: an analysis of products available in Brazil. **Rev Bras Ginecol Obstet**, v. 29, n. 5, p. 267 - 275, 2007.

TREMBLY A. Recent developments in calcium-related obesity research. **Obesity Reviews**, v. 9, p. 428-445, 2008.

TROINA AA, FIGUEIREDO MS, PASSOS MCF, REIS AM, ; OLIVEIRA E. ; LISBOA PC, MOURA EG. Flaxseed bioactive compounds change milk, hormonal and biochemical parameters of dams and offspring during lactation. **Food and Chemical Toxicology**, v. 50, p. 2388-2396, 2012.

TROWMAN R, DUMVILLE JC, HAHN S, TORGERSON DJ. A systematic review of the effects of calcium supplementation on body weight. **British Journal of Nutrition**, v. 95, p. 1033-1038, 2006.

TURKETZ H, GEYIKOGLU F, MOKHTAR YI, TOGAR B. Eicosapentaenoic acid protects against 2,3,7,8 tetrachlorodibenzo-p-dioxin-induced hepatic toxicity in cultured rat hepatocytes. **Cytotechnol**, 2012.

WASSON GR, MCKELVEY-MARTIN VJ, DOWNES CS. . The use of the comet assay in the study of human nutrition and cancer. **Mutagenesis**, v. 23, p. 153-162, 2008.

WILLIAN DL. Sugar Alcohols as bulk sweeteners. **Annu Rev Nutr**, v 9, p. 161-186, 1989.

WITT JSGZ, SCHNEIDER AP. Esthetic nutrition: body and beauty enhancement through nutritional care. **Ciênc. saùde colet**, v. 16, n. 9, p. 3909-3916, 2011.

YANOVSKI JA, PARIKH JS, YANOFF LB, DENKINGER IB, CALIS KA, REYNOLDS JC, SEBRING NG, MCHUGH T. Effects of Calcium Supplementation on Body Weight and Adiposity in Overweight and Obese Adults. **Ann Intern Med**, v. 150, p. 821-829, 2009.

ZANOBINI A, FFIRENZUOLI AM, TREVES C, BIANCHI A, CASEY H, BACCARI V. Influence of dietary sorbitol on the redox state of coenzymes and substrates linked to carbohydrate metabolism. **Pharmacol Res Commun**, v. 11, n. 4, p. 357-363, apr., 1979.

ZEMEL MB. Mechanisms of dietary modulation of adiposity. **J Nutr**, v. 133, p. 252- 256, 2003.

ZEMEL MB, RICHARDS J, MILSTEAD A, CAMPELL P. Effects of calcium and dairy on body composition and weight loss in African-American adults. **Obes. Res**, v. 13, p. 12181225, 2005.

ZEMEL MB, SHI H, GREER B, DIRIENZI D, ZEMEL P. Regulation of adiposity by dietary calcium. **FASEB J**, v. 14, p. 1132-1138, 2000.

ZEMEL MB, THOMPSON W, MILSTEAD A, MORRIS K, CAMPELL P. Calcium and dairy acceleration of weight and fat loss during energy restriction in obese adults. **Obes. Res**, v. 12, p. 582-590, 2004.

8. ANNEX 1

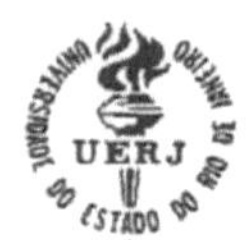

UNIVERSIDADE DO ESTADO DO RIO DE JANEIRO

INSTITUTO DE BIOLOGIA ROBERTO ALCANTARA GOMES

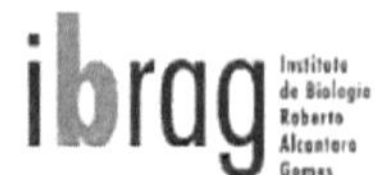

ETHICS COMMITTEE FOR THE CARE AND USE OF EXPERIMENTAL ANIMALS

CERTIFICATE

We certify that Protocol n^0 **CEUA/064/2012** on **"Effects of maternal consumption of sorbitol during lactation on nutritional parameters and toxicological evaluation in hepatocytes and blood of Wistar rats"**, under the responsibility of **Israel Felzenszwalb**, is in accordance with the Ethical Principles in Animal Experimentation adopted by the Brazilian College of Animal Experimentation (COBEA), having been approved by the Ethics Committee for the Care and Use of Experimental Animals of the Roberto Alcantara Gomes Biology Institute of UERJ (CEUA)$_1$ on **03/12/2012.** This certificate expires on **03/12/2016.**

Rio de Janeiro, December 3, 2012.

Profa. Patricia Cristina Lisboa
CEUA/IBRAG/UERJ

Prof. Israel Felzenszwalb
CEUA/IBRAG/UERJ

Profª Dra. Patrícia Cristina Lisboa da Silva
Profª Adj. do Depto. Ciências Fisiológicas / IBRAG / UERJ
Matrícula 34765-8

/.ass

☎ (21) 2587-6488 / 2587-6109 - Fax (21) 2284-9748
biologia@uerj.br

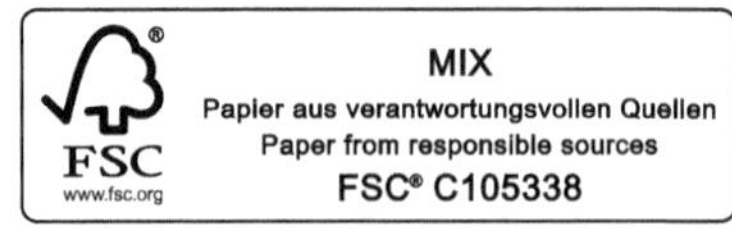

Printed by Books on Demand GmbH, Norderstedt / Germany